A 14-Day Ayur[...]
Lose Weight and Feel Your Best

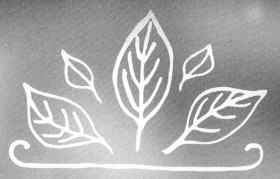

NEW YEAR
RE-SOLUTION

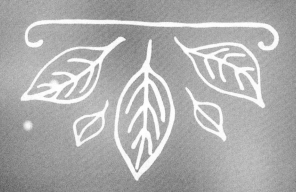

NOAH VOLZ

MW00959392

NEW YEAR
RE-SOLUTION

A 14-DAY AYURVEDIC PROGRAM TO
LOSE WEIGHT AND FEEL YOUR BEST

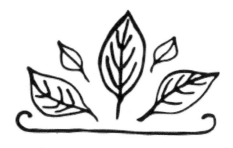

BY

NOAH VOLZ, CAS, LMT

RHYTHM OF HEALING

NEW YEAR RE-SOLUTION

A 14-Day Ayurvedic Program to Lose Weight and Feel Your Best

Copyright Noah Volz

ALL RIGHTS RESERVED

No part of this publication may be reproduced, stored in or introduced into a retrieval system, or transmitted, in any form or by any means (electronically, mechanical, photocopying, recording or otherwise), without the prior written permission of both the copyright owner and the publisher of this book.

Re-selling through electronic outlets (like Amazon, Barnes and Nobles or E-bay) without permission of the publisher is illegal and punishable by law.

The scanning, uploading, and distribution of this book via the Internet or via any other means without the permission of the publisher is illegal and punishable by law.

Please purchase only authorized editions and do not participate in or encourage electronic piracy of copyrightable materials.

Your support of the author's right is appreciated.

ISBN: 978-1-5196962-9-8

Cover Design: Octagon Labs

Interior Layout: ElfElm Publishing LLC

Disclaimer: This book is not intended to provide medical advice or to take the place of medical advice and treatment from your personal physicians. Readers are advised to consult their own doctors or other qualified health professionals regarding the treatment of medical conditions. The author shall not be held liable or responsible for any misunderstanding or misuse of the information contained in this manual or for any loss, damage, or injury caused or alleged to be caused directly or indirectly by any treatment, action, or application of any food or food source discussed in this electronic book. The statements in this book have not been evaluated by the U.S. Food and Drug Administration. This information is not intended to diagnose, treat, cure, or prevent any disease. competent jurisdiction. Both parties agree to pay their own attorney fees and costs, regardless of outcome, and the parties knowingly and voluntarily waive their rights to have their dispute tried and adjudicated by a judge or jury. The arbitration will take place in Fremont, CA.

Credits: All photographs were taken by Noah Volz and the graphic art was created by Octagon Labs and Elf Elm Publishing.

FOREWORD

AYURVEDA SPEAKS TO US FROM ACROSS THE CENTURIES, INVITING US to live a life more in pace and harmony with nature and the sacred: a saner, wiser, happier life. It invites us to slow down, relax, and rebuild. As someone who has worked with Ayurveda for more than thirty years in self care and healing, I appreciate the sustained and creative work that Noah Volz has put into this Re-Solution plan to reset one's approach to life and food. In this practical well-grounded program, he guides you through a month-long "reset" plan of action. Its goal is to enhance your protective essence (ojas), revitalize your digestive fire (agni), and increase the subtle vitality of prana, in order to re-invigorate your physical being. While doing so, you minimize ama, your toxic wastes, and the likelihood of disease. While its focus is on the wise use of resources to physically rejuvenate, this program also honors other aspects of your being – your need for spiritual renewal and to practically understand the research behind the methods. Rather than a heroic cleanse, this is an intriguing blend of purification and rejuvenation, a way to begin to create supportive habits for a lifetime, or a season.

The Re-Solution plan is set up in four simple stages. You get acclimatized to the idea that healing is possible in the Removal phase, letting go of some of your most life-sinking habits. In the Replacement phase, you begin to discover and use food tools for healthier living. The Repair phase gives you a chance to do a mini kind of Pancha Karma on your own, with delectable kichadis and healing teas. In the Re-innoculate/Post phase, you reintroduce the vitality of friendly microbes into your system, to recreate the roots of health within the gut so valued in Ayurveda.

If you're new to Ayurveda, Noah has a clear section about its principles and practices. If it's not new to you, it's easy to skip on to the Re-Solution plan.

The author uses accessible language and simple practical recommendations. He reminds us that to build ojas, we're going to need to schedule days so as not to hurry. He gives simple tips for lunch on the run and working with the American fascination for snacks. I especially appreciated Noah's innovative and nourishment packed recipes. Even if you do not choose to do the full program as it is laid out here, the recipes alone are great satisfying ways to sneak more veggies and whole foods into your life.

This program takes some planning; not everyone can thrive on it. Noah realistically warns his readers and potential participants that you'll need to invest an extra one to two hours per day on food prep until you've got the rhythm of it. You really do need to commit a full month to the process, if you wish to see its full effects. Yet for those readers who've wanted to do Pancha Karma on their own, who thrive on hands-on encounters with healing, who enjoy cooking and engaging in self care, this program could be a delightful and healing boon for you.

The herbs that are recommended here are high quality, organic, and respectful of the earth and its inhabitants. They are time-honored ways to purify and rejuvenate. Within the context of the author's experience, he has guided participants through this healing process with these specific herbs for nearly a decade. Yet Ayurveda is all about honoring individual differences and life conditions. Trust your own experience and common sense as you work with this plan, as well as the depth of the author's expertise. If you have an adverse reaction to a particular plant or food, do feel free to stop its use.* Inevitably, each of us has our own make up, and it is important to value this, as Ayurveda does.

At a time when it is easy to be swept into more and more day to day distractions that take us away from our true purpose and aims, Ayurveda invites us to ground and remember the sacred and the earth. You can respond to this nature-based invitation of healing in any way you choose, from letting go of your wi fi use for a day to clearing out the processed crud in your cabinets for a year, or making these delicious foods as often as you like. As you join Noah Volz in this adventure, may it benefit all sentient beings.

Amadea Morningstar
Santa Fe, NM
www.ayurvedapolarityyoga.com
October 30, 2015

*For example, shilijit is a highly effective remedy, especially for a person living in a moist climate. If you live in a different, drier, place, it may or may not suit your systems.

ACKNOWLEDGMENTS

I HAVE SO MUCH GRATITUDE AND THERE ARE SO MANY PEOPLE TO thank for the completion of this book. The initial idea for this book started in 2006 when I was working with Kimberly Ulrich at Ashland Ayurveda. Our collaboration generated a six week home pancha karma program that we facilitated together for many years to come. It was through this process that I started to recognize how Ayurvedic principles could be applied effectively to our modern world.

During this time was doing a lot of research in Ayurveda and K.P. Khalsa was extremely generous with his work sending me many articles and supporting my quest for knowledge. His expertise in herbalism and detoxification therapies were invaluable as I continued to create this program.

I would also like to thank Dr. John Douillard, even though I did not work with him one on one as I did my other inspirations it was the Colorado Cleanse that he created that would eventually provide the framework for the New Year Re-Solution program. His expertise in designing Ayurvedic programs for the modern world was exactly what I needed when the program was much longer and more complicated.

Additional recommendations and inspiration was received from Dr. Scott Blossom and the DoctorBlossom.com team. Through their expertise I was able to refine the program further until it became what it is today.

Ultimately it is the patients and students who have been undergoing the New Year Re-Solution program and its earlier iterations since 2006 that are the primary inspiration. My gratitude for their willingness to trust me to guide them through this process and to provide feedback is the most powerful reward of this creation. It is to them that I dedicate this work in the hopes that it will touch more lives of those who need it most.

Once the content was created there were many people along the way to help me finalize the manuscript and who gave me the confidence to share this with the world. The short list is my editor: Ann Maynard, my inspiration: James Altucher and the teams at ElfElm Publishing and Octagon Labs. Thank you for making this work a reality.

Noah Volz

Contents

NEW YEAR
RE-SOLUTION

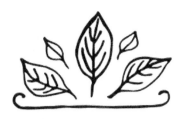

WHY RE-SOLUTION?

RE-SOLUTION IS NOT A DIET. IT'S NOT DEPRIVATION AND IT'S NOT FASTING. It is an opportunity to rid the body of foods and chemicals that you may be allergic to, and to improve the body's ability to dispose of toxic substances such as:

- Pesticides[1]
- Plastics[2,3,4]
- Phthalates and parabens in skin and hair care products[5]
- Solvents from paints
- Hormone disruptors found in city water[6]
- Internal waste that hasn't been eliminated

In Ayurveda (traditional Indian medicine) these varied substances are referred to as "*ama*" and their accumulation determines the disease process and how easy it is to resolve. The primary way *ama* accumulates is through dietary patterns that overwhelm the digestive fire and throw physiology out of balance. This can be overeating, eating inappropriate kinds or types of foods, or not taking enough time to eat. The Re-solution program prevents the accumulation of *ama* (and the habits that support it) through the removal of certain foods, taking herbs and performing certain lifestyle practices.[7] By committing yourself to this seasonal Re-solution, you will allow your body's detoxification machinery, which may be overburdened or compromised, to recover and begin to function efficiently again. This leads to increased energy, a feeling of lightness, sharpened senses, and the preservation of health over the long term.[8,9,10,11]

With enough accumulation of toxins the human body (which, like the earth, is composed of 75% water) is no longer able to transport and distribute cellular nutrition on its waterways, leading to physical and emotional imbalances. These imbalances manifest in a specific way, represented by the three *Doshas*: *Vata, Pitta,* and *Kapha.* The *Doshas* show how the waterways are either flowing in the wrong direction (*Vata*), inflamed (*Pitta*) or stagnant (*Kapha*). Re-solution is a safe and effective method to control the over-accumulation of the *Doshas*.

Get insider access to additional content and resources here: http://www.rhythmofhealing.com/newyearre-solution.html

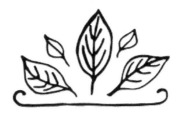

INTRODUCTION

DOES THIS SOUND EXCITING TO YOU? I AM NOAH VOLZ AND I HAVE BEEN practicing and teaching Ayurvedic medicine since 2006. During that time I have guided hundreds of people through the Re-solution program. I was sixteen when I was first introduced to yoga and healthy living. Although I followed a healthy lifestyle from that time forward I was not able to evade the wakeup call of disease. When I was twenty years old I had to drop out of college because I was bedridden for months first with strep throat, then with mononucleosis. It was clear that something had to change and it was during that time I was first introduced to Ayurveda. I healed my lungs through its gifts and was so profoundly changed that I started to read everything I could about it until I finally went to school to become a practitioner. What I love most about Ayurveda is that it is the premium prevention system for the modern world. The Re-solution program was born out of that love. The Re-Solution program is a reset button. It is a way to reboot your system so that you can allow healing to occur. With consistent effort and application the Re-solution program will change your life. But before we dive into the *How*, I want to talk about why this works and why it's important to your overall health.

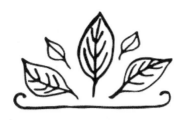

RE-SOLUTION AND CLEANSING

RE-SOLUTION AND CLEANSING ARE SIMILAR, BUT THEY ARE NOT THE same. Every bite we put in our mouth is both antioxidant and desirable (*sara*) or inflammatory and undesirable (*mala*). The digestive process ideally absorbs the *sara* to nourish the body and manages the *mala*. When the body is unable to adapt to the *mala* we begin to absorb wastes, which create more *ama* within the body.[12,13,14] This is how something may be healthy in a small amount but can become toxic (or *ama*-producing) in large amounts over time or in large quantities at a single meal. Or how some foods cause inflammation for some people and not for others. Re-solution inspires dietary and lifestyle habits that promote the removal of accumulated *ama* stored in the body and ignites the digestive fire. This is a cleansing response initiated from nutrition and lifestyle modifications, rather than fasting, deprivation or a long-term diet. What is common to both is that old patterns are replaced by new patterns that act as an investment in your overall health. It will take preparation, a little extra work, and a dedicated intention, but the result will be well worth it. By making a Re-solution today you are giving your future self the most valuable gift imaginable.

How it works

The Re-solution program works by addressing the three subtle *Doshas* of *Ojas*/Vitality, *Agni*/Digestive strength and *Prana*/Energy in order to minimize the amount of *ama* that is produced. The dietary recommendations provide high quality nutrition, but also give the digestive system a break. For example, eating 3 meals a day allows the digestive system the time and space it needs to fully digest the previous meal before the next one arrives. In a way the digestive system is like an assembly line and if there is not enough time between meals then the units on the line start to back up and causes *ama*. Vitality is supported by the lifestyle recommendations of going to bed early and reducing your commitments.[15] By slowing down and focusing on your experience during the program you will be able to replenish your stores of immunity and vitality. Lastly your energy levels are increased by doing yoga daily. You can use your own yoga routine or purchase the Yoga for Cleansing 3 DVD set on Amazon.

Why it Works

What makes the New Year Re-solution different than the many other programs that are out there is that it addresses body, mind and spirit through its focus on balancing the subtle *Doshas*.[16] As the subtle *Doshas* and their relative quantities determine health or disease of an individual this program does not focus on specific diseases. However it is effective for complaints such as:

- Fatigue and exhaustion
- Emotional immaturity and moodiness[17,18]
- Frequent colds and flues
- Body temperature fluctuations[19]
- Brain fog[20]
- Irritability
- Dry skin, hair loss and weight fluctuations
- Difficulty losing weight[21]
- Aching or painful joints
- Overall poor quality of life[22]

Ayurveda believes that experience is the best teacher, so don't take my word for it. Give the program a try and find out for yourself. But before you dive in I want to spend some time explaining the concepts that underlie Ayurveda.

FUNDAMENTALS OF AYURVEDA

IF YOU ARE ALREADY FAMILIAR WITH AYURVEDA FEEL FREE TO SKIP ahead to the Re-solution and Cleansing section. There are many exceptional books by amazing authors on the subject of Ayurveda. This will be a brief primer in order to help you understand the empirical and theoretical underpinnings of the Re-Solution program.

Over 5,000 years ago the medical practice of Ayurveda, literally "the science of life," was developed in order to address stress and disease in a both preventative and medical way. Although Ayurveda originated in India its methods and practice are uniquely relevant for our modern age as they teach us systems for living in harmony with natural rhythms. To understand how Ayurveda can help you. First we must dive into the elegant and practical features of *Prakriti* (individual's unique body/mind blueprint) and *Vikruti* (current imbalanced architecture).

Prakriti: Your Body/Mind Blueprint

Prakriti—your unique blueprint—is determined at the moment of conception and determines your inherited physical and emotional characteristics as well as your state of mind. In essence "form follows function." Like your genes your *Prakriti* is a blueprint of your unique characteristics such as height, eye color, natural hair color and innate personality traits. From the Ayurvedic perspective these inherent traits can be described simply through an understanding of the five elements and their qualities:

- Earth—heavy and dry
- Water—cold and wet
- Fire—hot and light
- Wind—light and dry
- Space—light

These qualities are relative to one another and it is through understanding the relative proportionality of each of these qualities throughout the body that will determine ones *Prakriti*. For example if you have more Earth you will have a large frame because it is associated with the heavy quality and larger individuals are heavier. If you have more Wind then you will have a lighter frame.

We are all different and unique and our body/mind blueprint reflects this individuality, but for the ease of categorization Ayurveda has identified three main types of blueprints that are easily distinguished from one another. These forces are called *Doshas.*

- *Vata*—Wind
- *Pitta*—Fire
- *Kapha*—Earth

The relative distribution of the *Doshas* makes you a unique individual. All three Dosha's are necessary and there is not one distribution that is better than another. However knowing your distribution can help you make decisions that are in alignment with your nature, leading to longevity and health.

For the sake of the blueprint model I will describe them in this way: *Kapha* is the plumbing and walls of the house, *Pitta* is the central heating unit and gas stove and *Vata* is the electricity in the house. Thus in every house (person) we have all three *Doshas*. Depending on how the house is built they are present in different ratios. For example, I may have the most *Pitta*/fire (a state of the art heating system), with a decent amount of *Kapha*/earth (a reasonably durable foundation, roof and walls) and only a small amount of *Vata*/air (minimal electricity, perhaps there are no lights), but someone else may have more *Vata* and *Pitta* and less *Kapha*. Just like every house is different with its own strengths and weaknesses, every individual is composed of unique strengths and weaknesses.

Knowing your body/mind blueprint is like knowing the original state of your house so that you have an awareness of its natural strengths and challenges. When you understand the blueprint you can take positive steps towards understanding our unique state of health. This allows you to connect deeply with the Source and be in alignment with your life's purpose. Without this awareness then any steps you take may not serve your unique nature.

Vikruti: Your Imbalanced Architecture

Understanding the current state of your house (architecture) and its need for maintenance is considered to be more important than the concept of *Prakriti* for the treatment of imbalances. *Vikruti*, as it is called, identifies how and where we have deviated from our natural, healthy and unique constitution. The word, *Vikruti* has the same root as the English words vicarious and vicissitudes, which both infer a negative change in the condition of body, mind and consciousness. This is your imbalanced architecture. If your body/mind blueprint, your natural or original state, is not maintained then the architecture or "complex and carefully designed structure" becomes imbalanced and leads to an unnatural or diseased state.

Your imbalanced architecture arises from the internal or external environment. This includes mental, emotional or physical stresses that increase *Vata*, *Pitta* and *Kapha* beyond their natural proportion of balance and adaptation. Thus excess in one or more of the *Doshas* leads to disturbances in the body and mind called *ama*. It is common for our internal state of mind to heavily influence the *Doshas* and that is why it is common for the *Prakriti* to become *Vikruti* over time. This imbalanced state will create an internal ecology where the body's natural self-corrective mechanisms are less able to do their job.

Back to the analogy of the house; *Prakriti* is our house and the walls and infrastructure of our body and mind are considered permanent characteristics. On the other hand temporary changes from daily stressors, *Vikruti*, create wear and tear that show up as fluctuations in weight, changes in mood, or developing a cough or runny nose, etc.

Primary Body/Mind Blueprints

Every individual's perspective and way that they relate to life is created by the unique proportion of the *Doshas* and the way they influence them. By understanding the underlying paradigm or the underlying blueprint by which you build your life you can create the life that serves you and those around you the most. The *Dosha's* define the way we interact and perceive the world. There are 3 primary *Doshas* that can combine to create 7 primary types. We will explore the primary tendencies of the three *Doshas* next.

Vata Types

As *Vata* is made of wind and space its qualities are dry, light, cool, rough, subtle and mobile. Some examples of how these qualities manifest in the body are in the table below:

Physiological

	Vata	Quality
Weather preference	Aversion to cold	Cold
Reaction to stress	Fear, uses energy to resolve stress	Mobile
Piggy bank	Impulsive, spends for pleasure	Subtle
Friendships	Makes friends easily, short term friends	Light
Activity Levels	High	Mobile

Physical

	Vata	Qualities
Hair amount	Thin	Light
Hair type	Dry	Dry
Skin	Dry, rough	Dry
Skin temperature	Cold hands/feet	Cold
Eyes	Small	Subtle
Size of teeth	Very large/small, crooked	Subtle
Weight	Thin, has trouble gaining weight	Light
Elimination	Hard, usually less than one bowel movement a day.	Dry
Frame	Small "delicate" frame and bone structure	Light
Chest	Flat chest	Light
Shoulders	Small shoulders	Light
Muscle	Lean muscle mass	Light
Metabolism	Fast metabolism	Mobile

No individual will have one hundred percent of these qualities so you are looking for those qualities that are high relative to the other two types and this will help you to optimize your diet and lifestyle to maintain balance in the midst of the gifts of these imperfections.

When there is an imbalance in one of these areas then moist, grounding, warming, smooth, oily and stabilizing foods and routines can be utilized.

Pitta Types

Pitta is predominantly associated with fire and some water which allows the qualities of oily, sharp, hot, light, malodorous, spreading and liquid to be present when there is a lot of *Pitta*. Here are some examples of what those qualities look like in the body:

Physiological

	Pitta	Quality
Hunger level	Needs food when hungry	Sharp
Sharing & giving	Large, infrequent giving	Spreading
Works best	Alone or as the leader of a group	Hot
Weather preference	Gets bloody noses or headaches with excess sunlight.	Hot
Reaction to stress	Anger, tries to control the situation.	Sharp
Piggy bank	Saves, big spender	Spreading
Friendships	Friends related to work or goals	Hot
Activity Levels	Extremely goal oriented	Spreading

Physical

	Pitta	Qualities
Hair amount	Loses hair easily	Heat
Hair type	Fine, oily	Oily
Eye size, shape	Deep set, medium	Liquid
Teeth	Yellows easily, red gums	Sharp
Weight	Gains muscle easily	Liquid
Elimination	Frequent, loose stools	Hot
Frame	Athletic	Spreading
Chest	Well defined chest	Sharp
Shoulders	Broad, wider than hips	Spreading
Muscle	Strong	Sharp
Metabolism	Gains/loses fat and muscle easily	Spreading
Body odor	Strong	Fleshy smelling

You probably noticed that you identified with some of the descriptions, but not all of them. It is not necessary to understand the *Dosha's* to be successful on the Re-solution program, but they can be a useful tool for maintaining health and managing acute diseases. This is because everything that exists inside and outside of the body can be explained by its dominant quality. In order to maintain the balance of *Pitta* dry, soft, cool, heavy, sweet smelling, and moderate interventions can be utilized.

Kapha Types

Kapha is composed of earth and water and its qualities are unctuous, cool, heavy, slow, smooth, soft and static. Sometimes dense, cloudy and viscous qualities are also included. Here are some examples below:

Physiological

	Kapha	Quality
Hunger level	Eats out of boredom or for flavor not necessity.	Heavy
Sharing & giving	Gives generously	Soft
Works best	In groups where they are told what to do.	Dense
Reaction to stress	Withdraws, utilizes the silent treatment	Heavy
Piggy bank	Saves regularly, miserly	Static
Friendships	Forms long lasting friendships	Smooth
Activity Levels	Low, needs motivation	Heavy

Physical

	Kapha	Qualities
Hair amount	Thick	Dense
Hair type	Oily	Unctuous
Skin	Thick skin, pale	Smooth
Skin temperature	Moist, cool, sometimes clammy	Cool
Eye size, shape	Large, big whites	Stable
Size of teeth	Large, white, few cavities	Dense
Weight	Large bones, sometimes overweight	Heavy
Elimination	Slow and steady	Smooth
Frame	Soft and pear shaped, big hips	Heavy
Chest	Large, barrel chested	Heavy
Shoulders	Short, stocky build. Broad, not as wide as hips	Static
Muscle	Round physique, not well defined	Heavy
Metabolism	Gains fat and muscle easily	Dense
Body odor	Sweet	Soft

Our uniqueness in how we respond to different foods and medicines can be explained through the Doshas. In order to maintain balance within a *Kapha* type warm, dry, light and stimulating foods and routines are utilized.

At the risk of oversimplifying things to make them available for a more general audience the three *Doshas* can be distilled into broader concepts called subtle *Doshas*. Unlike the *Doshas* that have a specific percentage that must be maintained, the subtle *Doshas* benefit by all being increased simultaneously. The overall goal of the Re-Solution program is to increase each one of the subtle *Doshas*, which relate to the *Doshas* in the following way.

- *Ojas = Kapha*
- *Agni = Pitta*
- *Prana = Vata*

Ojas: The Essence of Physical Form

Ojas is like the superhero version of the *Kapha Dosha* and is the most tangible of the subtle *Doshas* because it deals with the physical form. Every tissue in the body: lymph, blood, muscle, fat, bone and reproductive tissue has a relative strength and when these strengths are combined it creates our level of *Ojas*. *Ojas* is often measured by determining a person's stamina, endurance and vitality. If you have a lot of *Ojas* you will find that you can work 60–72 hour weeks and still be kind and generous to your loved ones. You will find that you can perform well in extreme sports and challenging athletic events. All activities that require a strong physical body. When the physical body starts to decline and injury becomes more prevalent or the skin and hair quality diminishes then more *Ojas* is being used then is being produced. Here are some simple suggestions for replenishing *Ojas*:

1. **Determine** what good digestion and a balanced diet means to you and follow your own advice.
2. **Incorporate** at least twenty minutes a day of contemplation, prayer or mediation.
3. **Mentally note** the proportion of optimistic to pessimistic feelings you have on a weekly basis and make a concerted effort to cultivate positive feelings, speech and behavior.
4. **Upon waking,** mentally list at least three things that you appreciate or are grateful for.
5. **Take** special Ayurvedic herbal formulations like those mentioned in "What to do after the Post phase."
6. **Schedule** your day so you don't have to hurry and if you find yourself hurrying let your mind slow down and become aware of the physical sensations associated with hurrying.

7. **Establish** a sleep routine that allows you to sleep through most of the night.

8. **Maintain** a level of physical activity and exercise that does not leave you feeling exhausted.

The Re-solution program is uniquely tailored in order to promote the production of *Ojas* in the body leading to long-term health.

Agni: The Fire That Transforms

We have all heard the old maxim, "you are what you eat." In Ayurveda this maxim is changed slightly into, "you are what you digest." The creation of *Ojas* is dependent on our ability to digest. Just as the creation of our body is dependent on digestion of what we eat. The key difference is that *Ojas* does not just transform food it is also the alchemical process that transforms our emotions and experiences into the substance of our being. Digestion in Ayurveda is called *Agni* and every natural health care provider seems to agree that digestion is the key to health. Ayurveda has identified four primary types of digestion (*Agni)* that will determine the amount of *Ojas* and that is produced in the body. Imbalances in *Agni* can also increase the *Dosha*s, which can lead to disease. The Re-solution program acts to bring *Agni* back into a balanced and regular state.

THE FOUR TYPES OF AGNI

1. **Regular or Balanced Digestion (SamAgni)** is the corner-stone of good health. It creates satisfaction around meals, mental clarity and emotional stability. Like all things it is a combination of all the right ingredients for the unique and dynamic needs of the individual. The three areas that can be assessed to determine if digestion is balanced are:

   a. **Appetite:** the individual has few cravings and most of them are seasonal in nature. You enjoy food, but it does not rule your life. You are hungry when it is time to eat and easily enjoy 3–2 meals a day.

   b. **Digestion:** directly after eating and for up to four hours after eating you have a comfortable feeling of your body digesting accompanied by intestinal sounds that sounds like a baby cooing with joy.

c. **Elimination:** There are variations in elimination patterns based on individuals and so there is no gold standard when it comes to elimination. The basics of balanced elimination is that you have a bowel movement at least once a day and it's consistency and shape is similar to a banana.

2. **Sharp Digestion (*TiksnAgni*)** is similar to when you get food poisoning. In order for the body to swiftly eliminate the bacteria that doesn't belong, alkaline and acidic enzymatic secretions are increased and delivered through increased circulation. This in turn stimulates the immune system to contain and eliminate any impurities. When your digestion is consistently like this over a long period of time it leads to excess *Pitta* and depletes *Ojas*. The three identifiers of digestion are affected in the following ways when digestion is sharp:

a. **Appetite:** the individual has excessive hunger and cravings, especially for the sweet taste as it is cooling and the body has generated a lot of heat in the form of inflammation.

b. **Digestion:** you are prone to acid indigestion or you get a sour taste in your mouth after eating that can last up to four hours. Your body feels hot after eating and your heart rate increases.

c. **Elimination:** your elimination is loose and frequent. Stools are unformed or have a small circumference.

3. **Slow Digestion (*MandAgni*)** happens when you eat too much food. Think of how your body and mind felt after your last Thanksgiving dinner. Your digestion is like a fire, and slow digestion is when you put too many logs on the fire and they don't burn well leading to lots of smoke and very little heat. The mind is powerful,

however, and so even when you have no appetite at all you can convince yourself to eat one more piece of pie. This is why slow digestion can create a *Kapha* imbalance. Here are some examples of slow digestion:

a. **Appetite:** your appetite is low and you can easily eat only two meals a day, but unlike balanced digestion you tend to crave certain foods and will eat based on your cravings not because you are really hungry.

b. **Digestion:** because the flame of your digestion is low you will often get some gas, bloating or a feeling of sleepiness or heaviness after eating. If the flame is not out completely and you will over time be able to digest everything completely; but you may feel like it was a lot of work and you need to refuel. This is why this type of digestion tends to lead to excess weight.

c. **Elimination:** you will have at least one bowel movement a day and it is usually well formed. Sometimes there is a feeling that there is more in there that won't come out.

4. **Irregular Digestion (*VisamAgni*)** If you are having trouble deciding whether you have sharp or slow digestion because you tend to fluctuate between the descriptions for each one, chances are that you have irregular digestion. Irregular digestion is common in individuals who are out of touch with their bodies and need to re-connect with their appetite, digestion and elimination. This is the type of digestion pattern that responds best to the Re-solution program. This pattern of digestion leads to an increase in the *Vata Dosha* and a decrease in *Ojas*.

a. **Appetite:** you may have intense periods of hunger alternating with a lack of interest in food. You often eat out of boredom or may overeat on your favorite foods and not leave room for your meal. Irregular appetite often leads to grazing or snacking instead of eating true meals.

b. **Digestion:** directly after eating and for up to four hours after eating you often have intestinal bloating, gas or abdominal discomfort with lots of noises coming from the intestines.

c. **Elimination:** Your elimination fluctuates from less than once a day with dry hard stools to more than three times a day with loose stools.

Any of the digestion types that is not balanced leads to *ama*. *Ama* will create traffic jams in the intestines. This can lead to leaky gut and other serious digestive complaints. To build *Agni* you develop a balanced approach to food that is not overly restrictive or hedonistic. Consistent pursuit ensures your body will get what it needs for a gentle, gradual and even increase of *Ojas*. Just like a real fire, our digestive fire requires air in order to burn it's brightest. If we don't allow oxygen to feed the fire it goes out. In the body circulation delivers the oxygen to the digestive system. The concept of *Prana* is what determines how circulation is maintained in the body and it will be described next.

Prana: The Movement Underpinning Life

Although *Prana* is a powerful force in the digestive system that guides the enteric nervous system and peristalsis, it is pervasive throughout the entire body. *Prana* is considered to be the foundation of the physical body in the same way that atoms and molecules are the foundation of all organic and inorganic matter. Because of the makeup of matter it abides by certain physical laws. In Ayurveda *Prana* are the laws by which the body maintains order. One way in which to understand *Prana* is as the force that is responsible for all the involuntary movement within the body. The enteric nervous system which is the gut's brain works on a subconscious level to give the body information about the needs of the digestive system. The brain is like the modem converting information into signals that can be used by the body and the enteric nervous system is like the router that connects to each individual organ. When there is a break in the flow of information between those three pieces then we must troubleshoot to find out where the problem is. The Re-solution program will provide the information about which lifestyle practices are adversely affecting your *Prana* and thereby hindering the subconscious functions of the digestive system leading to imbalance or disease.

The overall goal of the Re-solution program is to increase each of the characteristics of *Ojas*, *Agni* and *Prana* that help to strengthen and invigorate the body. As each of the subtle *Doshas* depend on each other the program helps the winds of *Prana* to blow on the fires of *Agni* to produce the nectar of *Ojas,* leading to long term health.

The Yin and Yang of Ayurveda

Restoration vs. Demolition

Chinese medicine and Ayurveda have long identified that there are two fundamental and opposing forces that invigorate and nourish life. *Brahmana,* or *Ojas,* is nourishing, cool, dark, slow, soft, stable, moist and tranquil. *Langana,* or *Agni,* is lightening, hot, bright, fast, mobile, dry and energetic. It is responsible for motivation, metabolism, transformation and active functions. It is reducing and in excess it can use up bodily reserves. *Ojas* is nourishing and builds the fluids and calms the mind. These are the primary principles that determine how a treatment is best administered. When there is an increase in the *Doshas* that creates "Imbalanced Architecture" this will lead to an excess or deficiency. Excess creates stagnation or an inability to detoxify adequately, and deficiency is when there is a lack of energy to nourish the system.

There are two primary Ayurvedic methods that treat these conditions: purification and rejuvenation. Rejuvenation is a form of restoration that acts to build the system and increases the fundamental *Ojas* of the body and mind. Purification is the primary form of lightening therapy and removes stagnation through detoxification and demolition by increasing *Agni*. Restoration is primarily used to pacify the increased *Doshas* by building the bodies innate energy supplies whereas demolition forcibly expels toxins and stagnation from the body. Every therapy can be evaluated in terms of whether it is restorative (building depleted reserves) or purifying (removing excess from the body). The Re-solution program combines both approaches. That is what makes this program so unique. Excess purification can lead to weakness and excess rejuvenation can lead to stagnation. The Re-solution program combines the best of both approaches in a way that allows both deficiency and excess to be resolved. In Ayurveda this is called "palliation," which is defined as "to relieve or lessen without curing; mitigate; alleviate." It is not a cure it is a Re-Solution!

Why Do the Re-Solution

For many of us, health is merely a means to an end and not an end in of itself. The Re-solution program is meant to be simple and effective. If you feel like the program is too heroic, then you may need to modify it so that it saves you energy instead of taking a lot of effort. The reason to do the Re-solution program may be health, but the ultimate aim is to plant the seed of some long term habits. It is unlikely that you will implement everything provided in this program, but if you make one lasting change then the program has been successful. Do your best and remember this program has the long term in mind and as you make it part of your New Year's routines you will learn a lot about yourself and make long-standing changes that will lead to more happiness in your life. That is the ultimate goal and health is merely a path towards improved happiness.

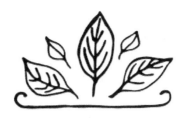

DAILY GUIDELINES FOR HEALTHY LIVING

Morning Routine

- Wake between 5:30–6:00 a.m. or earlier if your life requires it. Consider meditating upon arising.
- Milk or gently scrape your tongue per instructions provided.
- Drink 8–16 ounces of warm water.
- Perform your warm oil self-massage and steam, bathe or shower (refer to appendix for additional information on Abhyanga). At the end of your morning shower, give yourself a quick rinse with cold or lukewarm water. This flushes heat from the internal organs.
- Exercise for at least 30 minutes (walking, yoga, etc.) to get the blood and the lymph fluid circulating. Be gentle and breathe through the nose to keep your nervous system calm.

Mid-Day Routine

- Drink up to 4 cups of digestive tea (see appendix) a day.
- Make lunch your largest meal of the day and eat it between 12:00–2:00 p.m. Ensure that you feel satisfied with what and how much you eat in order to maintain a feeling of calm.
- After lunch, consider resting or taking a 10-minute walk outside to aid digestion before returning to work.
- In the afternoon, do 10–20 minutes of guided relaxation, meditation or breathing practices.

Evening Routine

- One hour after dinner, or before bed, take 2 tablets of Triphala to help with elimination.
- Recapitulation: Write down or reflect on your day and how you interact with people in your life.
- Turn off any flashing "rectangles" (T.V., phone, computer, etc.) after 7:30 pm.
- It will be most beneficial if you go to bed by 10:00 pm.

Note: Many of the morning routines can be done at other times of the day, but try to include all the recommended daily guidelines before you go to sleep at night.

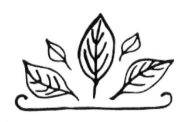

AHARA: GENERAL DIETARY RECOMMENDATIONS

THIS LIST IS BROKEN UP INTO THREE CATEGORIES. THE FIRST SECTION lists the foods, fats, herbs, and spices that will make up the bulk of your diet during the Re-solution. The second and third sections are comprised of foods that should only be consumed in small amounts and foods to be avoided during this time respectively.

Prioritize These Foods

Vegetables (buy local and organic)[26,27,28,29]

Broccoli

Brussel sprouts

Burdock

Cabbage

Cauliflower

Celeriac

Celery

Cabbage

Artichoke

Cucumber

Fennel

Seaweed

Jerusalem artichokes

All leafy greens

Kohlrabi

Leeks

Mushrooms

Onions, all types

Avocado

Parsnips

Peppers

Radishes

Sea veggies

Squash

Sweet potatoes

Turnips

Winter squash

Watercress

Seeds (and their butters and milks)—try sprouted or soaked for improved digestion

Chia	Sesame
Flax	Sunflower
Pumpkin	Hemp

Beans/Legumes[30]

Aduki	Mung
Black	Pinto
Lentils	Red

Fats/Oils[31,32]

Extra virgin sesame oil: low-medium heat, 350F/175C

Extra virgin coconut oil (not copra): low medium heat, 350F/175C

Extra virgin olive oil: medium heat, 405F/210C

Extra virgin almond oil: medium heat, 420F/216C

Organic palm and palm kernel oil: medium heat, 455F/235C

Organic grass fed ghee: high heat, 485F/252C

Extra virgin avocado oil: high heat, 520F/271C

All Raw, Unpasteurized Fermented Foods[33]

Krauts	Coconut kefir
Kimchee	Kombucha or jun made with-
Miso	out fruit juice
Pickles	

Sea Salt with High Mineral Content

Celtic

Himalayan

Hawaiian Red

Coconut Products (combine with ginger or other spices to improve digestion)

Butter

Milk

Oil

Herbs and Spices[34]

Ginger	Turmeric
Garlic	Fenugreek
Cilantro	Chili powder
Cumin	Curry powder
Coriander	Italian seasoning
Fennel	Basil
Cinnamon	Rosemary
Nutmeg	Tarragon
Cardamom	Oregano

Only Eat Small Amounts of These Foods

Carrots

Eggplant

Potatoes (white or red)

Tomatoes

Raw honey

Miso

Tempeh

Apples

Dried cranberries
     (if fruit-sweetened)

Pear

Avoid These Foods

All food additives and artificial sweeteners[35]

All processed or packaged foods[36]

All fried foods and trans fats[37]

Animal protein (broths made from bones are fine)

Coffee

Dairy (except as Takra)

Cereal grains

Sugar and all commercial sweeteners

Soy (except fermented soy: miso, tamari & tempeh in small
     amounts)

Glutinous grains, including wheat, spelt, kamut, rye, oats,
     barley[38,39,40]

Processed sugars and sweeteners

Caffeine in all forms including chocolate (matcha green tea is okay
     in moderation)[42]

Most non-organic foods.

How to Eat

- Eat until you are 75% full. One-third food, one-third water, one-third space.
- Eat three meals a day with no snacking.
- Eat after previous food is digested (3–6 hours). Usually equals three meals a day.
- Set a specific time and place for meals. Be consistent.
- Eat with proper frame of mind (a happy mood).
- Create a pleasant environment (flowers, music, and incense).
- Wash hands thoroughly prior to eating.
- Bless your food before eating.
- Take your time and chew your food longer, as it starts digesting in the mouth. If we enjoy the taste of food in the mouth it reduces the amount of food we eat.

How to Prepare for a Successful Re-Solution for Health

Plan your meals ahead of time. Anticipate that eating an elimination diet will take (on average) 1–2 more hours of food preparation time until you are used to this approach. Make a schedule of what you will be eating when. Make sure that you have adequate time in your day to be able to have the food that you need so that you don't feel stressed. Consider using kitchen gadgets such as:

- **Stainless steel rice cooker:** A rice cooker can save you time. After placing the ingredients for your Kitchari or a similar dish in the rice cooker with adequate water, you can flip the switch and it will cook to perfection and stay warm until you are ready for it. When using rice cookers make sure the interior is stainless steel and not aluminum. This is because high levels of aluminum exposure have been linked to neurotoxicity.[23,24]

- **Crock-Pot:** Make sure you have a high quality Crock Pot made of stainless steel or lead-free ceramics. (Most Crock-Pots made in China have lead in the glaze.)[25] You can place all the ingredients for a nourishing soup in a Crock-Pot and let it stew throughout the morning or afternoon so that you will have a warm nourishing meal when you are ready for it.

- **Thermos flask:** Most 12–15 hour stainless steel thermos's can be used to finish cooking a meal. After you bring your rice and beans to a boil, you can put the hot soup into a thermos with your spices and vegetables and eat the cooked beans and grains six hours later. This is a great option for lunch on the run.

Reduce your caffeine intake. Cut back on caffeine in the weeks and days before you begin. For example: if you drink two or more cups of coffee every day, ease back to just one; and then switch to half-caf;

then decaf, mate, or black tea. If you are a light coffee drinker, switch to green tea and then to herbal teas. The goal is to only drink herbal teas and water during the two weeks of your Re-solution.

Tell your family and friends. During the month, you'll eat specific meals; make time each day for asana, meditation, and other practices; and generally slow things down. See the resources section for suggestions of meditation and asana programs. Let the people in your life know about your plans beforehand so they can support you. Who knows? You may even convince a buddy or two to join you.

Cut your schedule back. A major reason for Re-solution is to reduce the amount of stress in your life. So, before the big day, look at your schedule and see where you can make some space. Cut out all non-essential commitments, even though it may mean saying "no" to some activities. Remember, you only have to shift things for a month but by doing so you'll be getting the most out of this process.

Stock your kitchen and get cooking. Make sure you have everything you need to prepare the foods in advance. Using the meal plans provided or make your own. You might even try making some of the recipes before the cleanse starts so that you're ready when the time comes.

Adjust your sleep schedule. During the two weeks of your Re-solution, try to get to sleep by 10:00 p.m. and wake up between 5:30–6:00 a.m. This schedule supports optimal liver function, provides ample rest, and will give you enough time to do some yoga and meditation before you start your day.

Set your intentions. This is a great opportunity to reflect on your life and how an Ayurvedic lifestyle might support you in realizing your goals and aspirations. Take time to define and refine your intentions for going through this process. These intentions will catalyze powerful energies of resolve and commitment within you.

General Home Wellness Guidelines

Follow these Guidelines during the two weeks of the program and for two weeks afterwards.

TAKE HERBS BEFORE AND AFTER MEALS

Before Meals — Take these herbs with water up to 15 minutes before meals.

- Banyan Botanicals Sweet Ease: Take 1 tablet, 3x/day, 15 minutes before meals with warm water.
- Banyan Botanicals *Pitta* Digest or *Kapha* Digest: Take 1 tablet, 3x/day, 15 minutes before meals with warm water.

After Meals — Take these herbs with an 8-ounce glass of water up to 15 minutes after meals.

- Banyan Botanicals Kidney Formula: Take 1 tablet, 3x/day, after meals for 4 weeks.
- Banyan Botanicals Immune Support: Take 1 tablet, 3x/day, after meals for 4 weeks.
- Banyan Botanicals Turmeric Tablets: Take 1 tablet 3x/day after meals for 4 weeks.
- Banyan Botanicals Shilajit Tablets: Take 1 tablet, 3x/day, after meals for 4 weeks.

Before Bed — Take these herbs before bed with 4 ounces of water.

- Banyan Botanicals Triphala Tablets: Take 2 tablets each evening.

Eat Three Meals A Day[42]

- Do not snack in between meals. If you absolutely need something, have fruit.
- If you are not used to eating three meals a day, start with four or five and work your way towards three meals a day.

Get Hydrated

- Hydration therapy: Sip hot water every 15 minutes throughout the day.
- Drink half your body weight in ounces of filtered pure, fresh water. (If you weigh 200 pounds then you would drink 100 ounces.)

Perform Ayurvedic Self-Massage with Oil

- Perform the short daily oil massage before you shower. See the Resources section for more information on how to do this.

Follow an Elimination Diet

- Reduce or eliminate intake of boxed, canned and packaged foods. Avoid sugar, alcohol, caffeine, chocolate, soy, wheat/gluten, meat, nuts and corn. Focus on eating whole foods that are organic, seasonal, colorful and fermented.

Practice Mindfulness

- Engage in yoga, breath work, and meditation daily.[43] See the Appendix for suggestions.

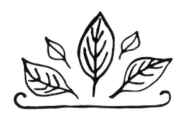

USING HERBS TO MAXIMIZE YOUR BENEFITS

THE FOLLOWING HERBS CAN BE PURCHASED ONLINE AT BANYAN BOTAN-icals. Please check out the Resources section for more information. When it comes to choosing herbs there are a plethora of different options that I could have chosen. I chose these specific herbs because they fulfill three criteria:

1. They are high quality, organic herbs cultivated with a focus on fair trade and sustainability.
2. They are Ayurvedic herbs and have been used in conjunction with detoxification programs for thousands of years.
3. They have been used successfully by my patients since 2006 with minimal side effects and maximum side benefits.

Increase Digestive Strength

Choose one of these formula's depending on the strength of your digestion. If you identified more with the Kapha descriptions and can tolerate spicy food well then choose Kapha digest. If you have a tendency towards heartburn or acid digestion or just want to use a gentler formula choose the Pitta digest.

BANYAN BOTANICALS PITTA DIGEST

Ingredients: Organic Guduchi, Amalaki, Cumin, Coriander, Fennel, Ajamoda, Licorice, Cardamom, Cinnamon bark.

This formula can increase absorption and is designed to support and enhance digestion, adrenal, spleen, and liver function, as well as reduce inflammation. It restores and regenerates the system by building healthy blood. It is cool in nature, with heat and toxin-clearing properties.

BANYAN BOTANICALS KAPHA DIGEST

Ingredients: Organic: Ginger, Black Pepper, Pippali.

This herbal compound activates cellular mechanisms to improve metabolic efficiency. Its ingredients can encourage optimal metabolic tissue and cellular responses and initiate the removal of invading pathogens and environmental stressors. It supports the body's natural internal defenses.

Lymphatic Detox and Adrenal Support

BANYAN BOTANICALS KIDNEY FORMULA

Ingredients: Gokshura, Punarnava, Guduchi, Manjista, Musta, Anantamul, Passionflower, Amalaki, Bibhitaki, Haritaki, Coriander, Fennel.

Stressors can cause many cells to become vulnerable to damage as time goes by, leading to inflammation, injured blood vessels, reduced oxygen supply, and low immune function. The antioxidants in Kidney Formula inhibit these degenerative changes, thereby normalizing gene behavior and decelerating adrenal fatigue.

TURMERIC

This herb has powerful modulators of prostaglandin and thromboxane activity, which are associated with inflammation. By improving the cell's response to inputs, further degradation is stalled and the cell begins to function in the optimum range.[44]

Balance Blood Sugar

BANYAN BOTANICALS SWEET EASE

Ingredients: Organic: Guduchi, Amalaki, Shardunika, Turmeric, Arjuna, Neem.

Ingredients in Sweet Ease affect physiological function by altering metabolic pathways and directing the utilization of key nutrients necessary for maintaining proper blood sugar and insulin levels. This provides the structural framework for efficient energy utilization and storage.[45,46]

Thin the Bile and Improve Immune Function

BANYAN BOTANICALS IMMUNE SUPPORT

Organic: Licorice, Kalmegh, Pippali, Turmeric, Ginger, Echinacea, Osha, Amalaki, Bibhitaki, Haritaki, Black Pepper, Cardamom.

Endogenous toxins and exogenous toxins can cause cellular damage, compromise immune function and promote hormonal imbalance. As a primary organ of detoxification, the liver being is designed to remove toxins from cells through a series of enzymatic reactions. When this system doesn't function properly (and there is toxic build up), Immune Support can help by supporting healthy activity of detoxification enzymes within the liver and body.

Boost Absorption, Mood and Energy

BANYAN BOTANICALS SHILAJIT (HIMALAYAN MINERAL PITCH)

The body's capacity to detoxify and preserve its equilibrium in response to constant and inexorable fluctuations has defined limits. If that capacity is exceeded, our ability to maintain an optimal state of health is compromised. Shilijit increases our ability to cope with stress, balance hormones, build stamina, assist in glucose control, and support faster recovery from injury.[47,48,49]

Improve Elimination

BANYAN BOTANICALS TRIPHALA

Ingredients: Organic: Amalaki, Bibhitaki, Haritaki.

Triphala is a rich source of polyphenols, which are regarded as highly potent antioxidants. One of them —ellagic acid—has been well researched and proven to be an effective free radical scavenger that eliminates toxins in the body, thereby protecting cells (including those in the brain) from their damaging effects.

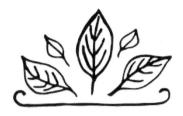

MONITORING THE TONGUE

MONITORING THE TONGUE IS A VERY IMPORTANT THING TO DO DURING this process. It reflects the state of the digestive system and will provide information on how the cleanse is affecting your internal organs. Look for a slight coating on the tongue. If the coating is getting thicker, the foods that you are choosing and the amount you are eating are not supporting the Re-solution and could be changed to improve your results. In order to monitor the tongue, use one of the two methods listed below.

Tongue Milking

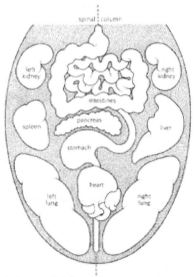

Note: This diagram is used to look at one's own tongue in a mirror. It is a mirror image.

First, purchase three washcloths that have a look and texture you like. These will be used solely for the purpose of cleansing your tongue. The tongue is considered to be a map of the digestive system. The upper thoracic cavity and the organs therein are found toward the tip of the tongue and the organs of the pelvic bowl are found at the root of the tongue. Overall, tension in the abdominal organs can be alleviated through the method of tongue milking.

During your early morning routine, before you eat or drink anything, take one corner of the washcloth and place it in the mouth. Pull it forward against the surface of your tongue; reverse the washcloth and repeat.

After the tongue surface has been cleaned, it is time to reduce the tension in the organs. This process must be done with awareness and attention.

Using the washcloth, take hold of the tongue with the fingers on both sides and stretch the tongue forward slightly, being careful not to cause any discomfort on the frenulum. Then drag the tongue to the left and to the right. Draw it up and draw it down (you may have to change your hand position). Then twist the tongue in both directions (left and right). After this process is complete, the tongue should feel loose and the corresponding organs should feel like they are floating within the abdominal cavity.

Tongue Scraping

Look at your tongue. Notice any variation of color, texture, coating, etc. This indicates how well you are digesting your food. Use a stainless steel tongue cleaner to **gently** scrape the tongue, and then wash the scraper to remove the buildup. Repeat 3–5 times or until very little build up is present when washing.

Hydration Therapy

Get a large stainless steel thermos (1 quart) and fill with boiled water. Let cool until it is warm/hot but drinkable. Sip 1–2 mouthfuls every 15 minutes throughout the day and refill as necessary. Make sure that you are drinking 8 to 12 glasses (8 ounces each) of water a day through this and other methods. One strategy is to drink 8 ounces of water for every two hours you are awake, starting with at least 2 8-ounce glasses of warm water in the morning before any food intake.

The Benefits of Drinking Water
- Water can dilute and eliminate toxic accumulations.
- Water detoxifies our skin, kidneys, and improves our ability to sweat during exercise.
- We lose 48 to 64 ounces of water a day through urination, sweating, and breathing.

The Importance of Drinking Water
- Fatigue and headaches can be remedied by adequate water consumption.
- Hunger is usually an indication of dehydration.
- When we are under-hydrated our metabolism slows down.
- Muscle and joint pain gets worse with dehydration.
- The brain depends on water. Our memory, concentration, and focus are all affected by water intake.

What Does Water Do?
- Improves absorption of vital nutrients.
- Transports nutrients to cells and tissues.
- Transports wastes to the kidneys for filtration and elimination.
- Retains and transports heat.

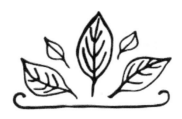

THE CLEANSE

Overview

REMOVE: Day 1–3, Removal Phase

- Follow General Wellness Guidelines.
- Follow Daily Guidelines for Healthy Living.
- Eat 1–2 handfuls of purple or blue foods (beets or berries).
- Drink one 8-ounce glass of Apple Cider Elixir.
- Drink lemon water

Supplies: Beets, blueberries, blackberries, elderberries, huckleberries, cherries, ginger, apple cider vinegar, lemon, Banyan herbal supplements, tongue cleaner or washcloths.

REPLACE: Day 4–7, Replacement Phase

- Do daily self-massage and steam or hot shower.
- Drink a Winter Elixir for breakfast.
- Eat at least four handfuls of veggies a day.
- Continue General Wellness Guidelines.
- Continue Daily Guidelines for Healthy Living.

Supplies: Liquid Stevia, coconut oil, ghee, and teas for the elixir. Mahanarayan oil for Abhyanga.

REPAIR: Day 8–11, Repair Phase

- Eat Kitchari for 3 meals each day, choosing the option that feels best for you.
- Increase your dose of after-meal herbs to 2 per meal.
- Continue General Wellness Guidelines.
- Continue Daily Guidelines for Healthy Living.

Supplies: Mung dahl, basmati rice or quinoa, spices, and vegetables.

REINNOCULATE: Day 12–14, Post Phase

- Eat 1–2 Tablespoons of kraut with every meal.
- Drink Takra before every meal.
- Eat probiotic rich foods like miso.
- Increase your dose of *Pitta/Kapha* digest.
- Continue General Wellness Guidelines.
- Continue Daily Guidelines for Healthy Living.

Supplies: Nancy's whole milk yogurt or greek yogurt, kraut and miso.

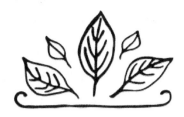

DAY 1–3 REMOVAL PHASE

THE REMOVAL PHASE IS DESIGNED TO STIMULATE THE PRODUCTION OF hydrochloric acid in the stomach and to liquefy the bile in the gallbladder to improve digestion of fats. Most of the hard to remove *ama* and toxins are stored in the fat cells making it difficult for you to lose weight. By using the apple cider vinegar elixir, lemon water and colorful foods you remove *ama* stored in the fat cells. This process wakes up *Agni* and begins the process of removing *ama* that is blocking the flow of *Prana* and depleting your energy as well as stopping *Ojas* from being produced.

Dietary Recommendations

- Follow the General Home Wellness Guidelines and Daily Guidelines for Healthy Living.
- Drink the 1–3 glasses of the Apple Cider Vinegar (ACV) Elixir.
- Drink 3 or more glasses of warm lemon water per day.
- Increase your intake blue, green and purple foods such as beets or berries such as blueberry, blackberry, raspberry, cranberry, cherry or pomegranate.
- In addition to the ACV elixirs and colorful foods, eat an elimination diet with an emphasis on vegetable soups, legumes and a light quantity of gluten-free grains.

Supplements & Beverage Recommendations

- Take 2 Triphala tablets in the evening before bed.
- Take 1 tablet of Sweet Ease and *Kapha* or *Pitta* digest before meals.
- Take 1 tablet of Kidney Formula, Immune Support, Turmeric and Shilajit between meals.
- Drink warm beverages, such as herbal tea, throughout the day.

Removal Phase Meal Suggestions

In order to find a meal system that works for you, start where you are. Look at your common breakfasts, lunches, and dinner and incorporate the lemon water, ACV elixir, and blue, green, and purple foods into your current routines. Below I have included a sample meal plan as a guide:

Sample Meal Plan for Removal Phase

Day	Breakfast	Snack	Lunch	Snack	Dinner
Day 1	Water with lemon. Grated beets, apples and spinach oatmeal with hemp milk	ACV Elixir	Salad with dressing of choice	ACV Elixir	Beet dahl soup with cilantro chutney
Day 2	Water with lemon. Beet zucchini pancakes with apple butter	ACV Elixir	Salad with dressing of choice	ACV Elixir	Wild rice salad
Day 3	Water with lemon. Savory chard and chia pudding	ACV Elixir	Salad with dressing of choice	ACV Elixir	Winter Root Veggie Soup

Removal Phase Recipes

While these recipes are intended as a guide, they do not need to be followed to the letter. Feel free to omit or add things to the recipes so that they fit your unique needs. In general the only rule to follow during this phase are the dietary recommendations listed above.

Note about recipes: I made money by cooking in high end restaurants all through high school and college. This means two things. One is that I never measure anything. I have created these recipes to the best of my knowledge based on what I think I would do, but I am always substituting what I have on hand for what is called for. The other thing that this means is that each recipe makes a lot of food. If you are a family of four then you may run out, but more than likely you will have more than you need. That is why it is nice to do this with a friend or invite people over for dinner when you are making these recipes.

ACV (APPLE CIDER VINEGAR) ELIXIR

Ingredients:

- 1 tablespoon raw, unpasteurized apple cider vinegar
- 5–7 drops of stevia (lemon flavored is my favorite)
- 10 ounces of water
- Optional: 2–4 ounces of aloe vera juice
- Pinch of powdered ginger

Directions:

Mix all ingredients and serve.

You can have up to 16 ounces a day.

You can make a large batch and shake and drink from it during the day.

Apple Cider Vinegar	Sēvama (Sanskrit)	Malus Domestica

Character: *The Decongester*
ACV improves circulation in the body and can remove emotional stagnation and bad moods. ACV has been used to remedy sluggish digestion or indigestion, and is even more powerful than lemon juice in this regard. The acid inhibits the growth of disease-producing bacteria and neutralizes poison.

Guna: warming **Rasa:** pungent, sour **Vipaka:** pungent **Virya:** warm **Prabhava:** gall stones	**Main Action:** Appetite stimulant, liver cleanser **Action on *Doshas*:** P+ VK- **Action on Dhatus:** Especially good for the lymph, blood and fat

Description:
Can be used to stimulate the gallbladder and softens gallstones, promoting liver health. It is detoxifying and can assist in the treatment of bacteria, fungus and candida. Apple cider vinegar is rich in natural minerals, vitamins, and enzymes. Taking apple cider vinegar before meals aids digestion and improves gastric health, boosting your body's ability to keep that stomach acid at is optimum. ACV can also relieve excess *Kapha* in form of edema, body weight, excess mucus or athlete's foot. The pectin is a form of fiber, which can remove cholesterol, heavy metals, lead, mercury, and radiation residues.

Apples can benefit the emotional depression associated with low blood sugar conditions.

Main Uses:
Gastritis, colitis, and burning infections
Gallbladder or liver congestion
Infections especially of viral origin

BEET AND SPINACH OATMEAL

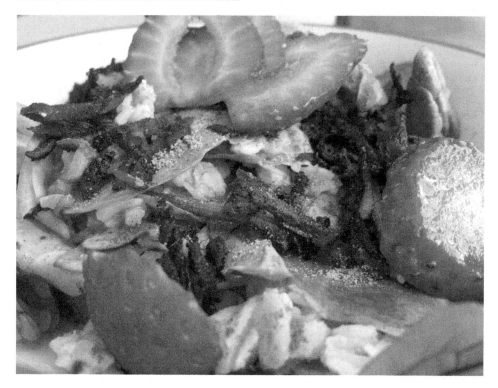

Fruit is best eaten by itself during this program. Although this photo includes strawberries it is best to not include them in the recipe.

Ingredients:

- 1 grated beet
- 1 handful spinach
- ¼ cup gluten-free rolled oats
- 1 teaspoon fresh ground flax seed
- 1 tablespoon coconut oil
- 1 tablespoon fresh minced ginger
- 1 teaspoon cinnamon
- 1 teaspoon cardamom
- 1 cup filtered water
- ¼ cup hemp or coconut milk

- Optional:
  - Chia seeds
  - Hemp seeds
  - 7 drops liquid stevia
  - Fennel powder

Directions:

Bring water to a boil and add all ingredients except for spinach and hemp milk.

Add more water if necessary and cook for 5–10 minutes, adding spinach at the very end.

Add hemp or coconut milk to cool and serve.

I usually grind a cup of flax at a time and store it in the refrigerator.

BEET ZUCCHINI PANCAKES

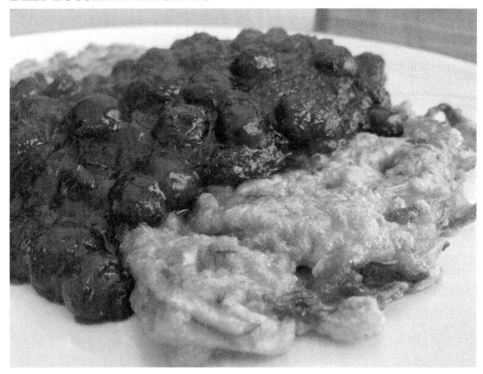

Ingredients:

- 1 grated beet
- 1 grated zucchini
- 1 cup shredded sweet potato
- 1 Tablespoon fresh ground flax seed
- ½ cup warm water
- 1 tablespoon coconut flour
- ½ teaspoon baking soda
- 1 teaspoon ground cinnamon
- 1/8 teaspoon ground or freshly grated nutmeg
- 1 tablespoon ghee
- Water to desired consistency

Directions:

Once you make these a few times you will find the consistency of batter that works the best.

Start by grating the beet, zucchini, sweet potato into a large bowl.

Then combine the flax meal with a ½ cup of warm water and let sit.

Add remaining ingredients except for ghee to the shredded veggies.

Heat a skillet on the stove and place ghee in it.

Then combine the flax and water with ingredients and stir until you have a thick batter. You may need to add more water.

Then scoop out about a ¼ cup of batter and pat it flat in the skillet. You may have to add more ghee as you go if things start to stick.

Fruit digests much faster than all other foods and when combined with other foods it can lead to fermentation in the stomach and small intestine creating an environment for bacterial overgrowth.

Although I have included fruit in the recipe for the sake of the picture it is best to cover your pancake in ghee or maple syrup instead of the berry coulis.

BERRY COULIS

Ingredients:

- 1 tablespoon psyllium husk powder
- 1 tablespoon fresh squeezed lemon juice
- 1 pint blueberries
- 5–7 drops liquid stevia
- 3 tablespoons water

Directions:

In a small bowl, whisk the psyllium in the lemon juice until dissolved. Set aside.

Place the blueberries, stevia and water in a small saucepan. Bring to a boil and simmer for 4 minutes.

Add the psyllium and lemon juice mixture and stir to combine. Simmer for another 3–4 minutes until blueberries are very soft and sauce has thickened.

Serve warm over pancakes or ice cream, or refrigerate up to 5 days for later use. Sauce will thicken as it sits and cools.

SAVORY CHARD AND CHIA PUDDING

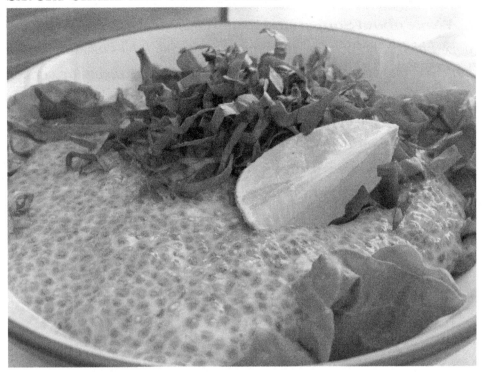

Ingredients:

- 2 cups hemp milk
- 3 tablespoons chia seeds
- 1 handful of red chard leaves, diced
- 1 tablespoon fresh basil leaf, chopped
- Splash of lime juice
- Pinch of black pepper
- 1 teaspoon fennel seed powder
- Optional: berries or cucumber slices
- Pinch of salt

Directions:

Soak chia in hemp milk overnight. Mix with remaining ingredients.

LUNCH AND DINNER

A Note about Soups: Most soups start with what is called a mire-poix which is French for roughly chopped vegetables usually including carrots, celery and onions. Every culture has a similar version and it is what makes their food so delicious. You can't go wrong by starting a recipe with these three ingredients. Here are a few other examples. Italian soffritto includes onions, garlic and tomato. German suppengrun is leeks, carrots and celeriac. Polish wloszczyzna is leeks, carrots, celery root and parsley root. The creole holy trinity is onions, celery and bell peppers. The French duxelles is shallots, mushrooms and butter.

CREAM OF WINTER ROOT VEGETABLE SOUP

Ingredients:

- 3 tablespoons ghee
- 2 onions, sliced
- 3 cloves garlic, chopped
- 2 parsnips, peeled and sliced
- 2 turnips, cubed
- 2 beets, peeled and sliced
- 1 cup celery root, peeled and cubed
- ½ head cabbage, sliced
- 2 Tablespoons peeled, chopped ginger
- 2–3 teaspoons dried thyme
- 5–6 cups vegetable broth
- 1 (13.5-oz) can coconut milk
- Salt and pepper to taste

Directions:

Place ghee in a large pot and add garlic, onions, parsnips, turnips, celery root and beets.

Sauté on medium heat for about 10 minutes, or until the roots start to soften.

Add cabbage, ginger, and thyme and stir until cabbage softens, about 5 minutes.

Then add water or vegetable broth to cover, and then can of coconut milk.

Cook until vegetables are soft. You may want to puree in a blender.

Beet Dahl

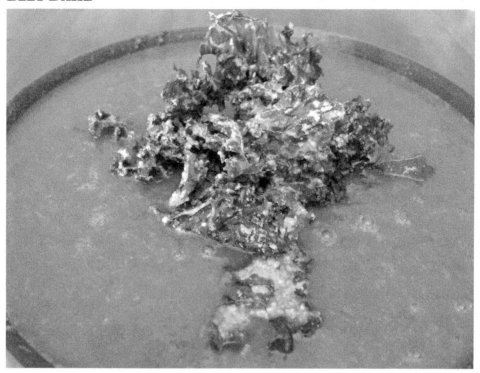

Ingredients:

- 1 cup red lentils or split mung beans
- 3 beets, cubed
- 1 yellow onion, diced
- 2 stalks celery, diced
- 2 carrots, diced
- 1 handful kale or spinach
- 1 teaspoon fennel powder
- 1 teaspoon curry powder
- ¼ teaspoon chili powder
- 1 teaspoon coriander
- ¼ teaspoon fenugreek
- ¼ teaspoon turmeric

- ¼ teaspoon cumin
- 2 tablespoons ghee
- Water
- Salt to taste

Directions:

Soak red lentils overnight. In a large soup pot, add diced onion to melted ghee and sauté.

After 5 minutes, add celery, carrots, and cubed beets.

Stir frequently and add more water if they stick to the bottom.

Add lentils and remaining ingredients except for the spinach or kale.

Add enough water or vegetable stock to cover ingredients (approximately 2 cups).

Bring to a boil and then turn heat to low.

Cook for 20–30 minutes or until lentils are soft, then add spinach.

Add salt to taste.

CILANTRO CHUTNEY

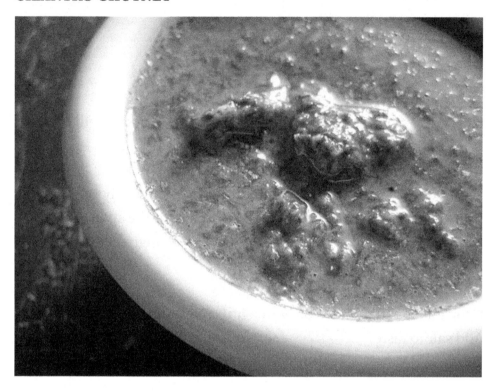

Ingredients:

- 1 bunch fresh cilantro
- ¼ cup fresh lemon juice
- ¼ cup water
- ¼ cup grated coconut
- 2 tablespoons fresh ginger root
- 1 medium-sized granny smith apple
- 1 teaspoon sea salt
- ¼ teaspoon fresh ground black pepper

Directions:

Blend all ingredients until roughly chopped. This can be stored for about one week in the refrigerator.

WILD RICE AND BEET SALAD

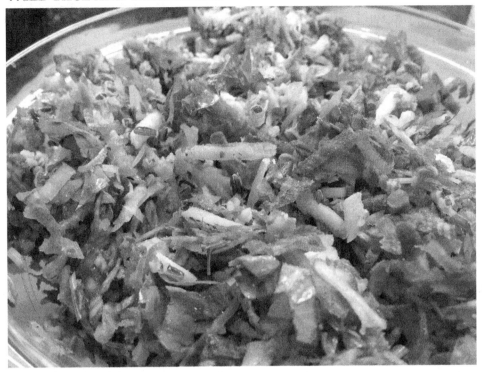

Ingredients:

- 1 cup wild rice, soaked for 8–16 hours and cooked
- 3 cups water
- ½ cup roasted pumpkin seeds
- 1 diced red pepper
- 1 grated medium-sized red beet
- 1 medium-sized grated apple
- 1 cup chopped parsley
- ½ cup small dice green onion

Directions:

Soaking the wild rice will decrease cooking times significantly. You will know the rice is done when the seeds split open.

Bring water and rice to a boil and then turn down heat and cook for 30–45 minutes.

When water has fully absorbed, add shredded red beets, red pepper, parsley, apple, green onion and toasted pumpkin seeds.

Toast pumpkin seeds lightly in a toaster oven, about 5 minutes.

When rice is cool add the remaining ingredients.

Dressing:

Ingredients:

- ◦ 1 tablespoon apple cider vinegar
- ◦ ¼ cup apple juice
- ◦ 2 tablespoons olive oil
- ◦ 1 tablespoons lemon juice
- ◦ 1 tablespoons mustard
- ◦ 1 teaspoon basil

Directions:

To make the dressing, mix all ingredients together and blend until oil and vinegar no longer separate.

LARGE SALAD WITH DRESSING OF CHOICE

Creamy Hemp Seed Dressing

Ingredients:

- ½ cup olive oil
- ¼ cup lemon juice
- 2 tablespoons wheat-free tamari
- ½ cup water
- ½ an avocado
- 1 tablespoon nutritional yeast
- 1 cup hemp seeds
- 1 inch piece of peeled ginger
- ¾ teaspoon salt
- ¼ teaspoon black pepper
- ¼ cup loosely packed fresh cilantro leaves

Directions:

Combine all ingredients in a high-speed blender and blend until smooth.

Sesame Miso Dressing

Ingredients:

- ½ cup water
- ½ cup sesame oil
- 2 ribs celery, chopped
- Juice of half a lemon
- 3 tablespoons wheat-free tamari
- 2 tablespoons chickpea or mellow white miso
- 1 tablespoon dulse flakes
- 1 tablespoon nutritional yeast
- 1 tablespoon honey

Directions:

Place all ingredients in a high-speed blender and blend until smooth. You can double or triple the recipe and store this in the refrigerator for about a week.

Note About the Removal Phase: *ACV and Lemon are extremely effective and removing ama in the form of bacteria, yeasts, fungus and undigested food. Long term and frequent use of these liquids can however weaken the teeth. If you really enjoy the ACV and lemon water make sure that you are not drinking them more than 4x's a week and take at least a week off after drinking them for a month in order to allow the body to remodel.*

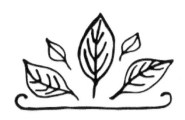

DAY 4–7 REPLACEMENT PHASE

AFTER THE REMOVAL PHASE IS COMPLETE, SHIFT YOUR FOCUS TO PRO-cedures that stabilize the system with high quality building blocks. "Nature abhors a vacuum." So as we remove the unwanted *ama* the body will search for a replacement. This is accomplished through the high quality fats in the elixirs. Fat cells are instrumental in balancing our hormone levels, and if the fat cells are clogged with *ama* we must first remove the *ama* and then reboot the fat cells in the replacement phase. You can continue to drink the ACV elixir, lemon water and eat colorful foods if you are inspired, but at this point they are not required. The replacement phase will use oil massage, elixirs and warm baths in order to allow high quality fatty acids to replace the toxic *ama* in the body so that the body does not try and hold onto the toxins when you transition into the Repair phase. This is the phase where you will start to reap the benefits of your work so far and prepare the mind for letting go of detrimental dietary habits and attachments.

Dietary and Beverage Recommendations

- Follow the General Home Wellness Guidelines and Daily Guidelines for Healthy Living.
- Drink 1 elixir of your choice in the morning. You may need to have breakfast a couple hours later.
- Follow the Hydration therapy by sipping warm water every 15 minutes to purify the lymph.
- Drink warm beverages, such as herbal tea, throughout the day.

Lifestyle Recommendations

- Perform warm oil massage on yourself or schedule and Ayurvedic massage.
- Take warm showers daily or warm baths, steam room or sauna for 30 minutes a day.

Elixir Recommendations

Day 4: Follow the recipe as indicated, including 1 Tablespoon of ghee and 1 Tablespoon of coconut oil.

Day 5: Stay at 1 Tablespoon each of ghee and 1 Tablespoon coconut oil.

Day 6: Increase amount of oil in elixir to 2 Tablespoons of ghee and 2 Tablespoons coconut oil.

Day 7: Stay at 2 Tablespoons of ghee and 2 Tablespoons coconut oil.

Note: *Elixir recommendations were inspired by Dave Asprey's work with Bulletproof coffee. Monitor your tongue closely on these days, as you don't want to overwhelm your digestive fire. If the coating on your tongue is increasing, decrease the amount of ghee and coconut oil you are using back to the dosage from the previous day.*

Supplements Recommendations

- Take 2 Triphala tablets in the evening before bed.
- Take 1 tablet of Sweet Ease and *Kapha/Pitta* Digest before meals.
- Take 1 tablet of Kidney Formula, Immune Support, Turmeric and Shilajit after meals.

Replacement Phase Meal Suggestions

Day	Breakfast	Lunch	Dinner
Day 4	Chai Elixir	Stuffed Delicata Squash	Carrot Ginger Soup with Steamed Kale
Day 5	Winter Elixir	Ginger Yam Soup with Steamed Kale	Butternut Squash Soup with Steamed Kale
Day 6	Magic Morning Elixir	Carrot Ginger Soup with Steamed Kale	Stuffed Delicata Squash
Day 7	Tension Tamer Elixir	Ginger Yam Soup with Steamed Kale	Butternut Squash Soup with Steamed Kale

Recipes for the Replacement Phase

Like the previous suggestions these recipes can be used as a guide. Feel free to omit or add things to the recipes so that they fit your unique constitution.

Note: *In traditional Ayurvedic cleansing patients are instructed to drink increasing dosages of ghee every morning. Ghee is used because it binds to fat soluble toxins and dampens the digestion so that the body is no longer focused on taking in nutrition, but instead of eliminating toxins. These procedure is extremely effective, but is best done with the guidance of skilled practitioner. The compromise is to use the elixirs. Elixirs are based on the work of Dave Asprey and Andrea Nakayama, both experts in their field. I have used their research to create these unique Ayurvedic elixirs. The emulsification of the oils with the hot beverage allows them to penetrate more deeply and to facilitate the removal of fat soluble toxins and to help the body receive the fat it needs to fight cravings.*

Chai Elixir

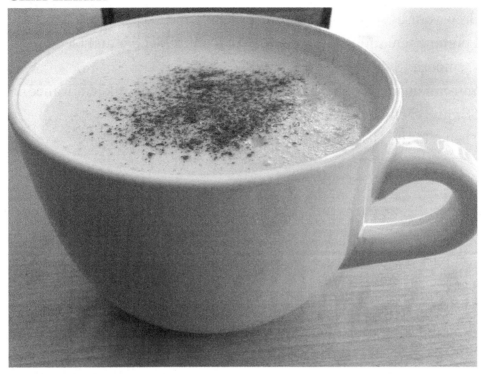

Ingredients:

- 2 bags of Rooibos Chai
- Hot water (8–16 ounces)
- Pinch of cardamom powder
- 7–10 drops vanilla crème liquid stevia
- 2–3 tablespoons coconut milk or nut milk
- 1–2 Tablespoons coconut oil
- 1–2 Tablespoons ghee
- Optional: 1 teaspoon Great Lakes unflavored gelatin or psyllium husk powder for a thicker texture.

Directions:

Brew your tea bags for 10 minutes. Strain and set aside.

Combine remaining ingredients with tea in a blender and blend until smooth.

You can quadruple the tea, cardamom, stevia and milk in advance.

Stir and then heat up a cup in a saucepan.

Then add the oils and blend.

WINTER ELIXIR

Ingredients:

- 1 teaspoon Ashwagandha or Maca powder
- ½ teaspoon cinnamon powder
- ¼ teaspoon ginger powder
- 1–2 Tablespoons coconut oil
- 1–2 Tablespoons ghee
- 2–4 Tablespoons Native Forest Coconut Milk
- Stevia to taste (5–7 drops)
- ½ cup hot water, or more to taste
- Optional: 1 teaspoon Great Lakes unflavored gelatin or psyllium husk powder for a thicker texture.

Directions:

Place all ingredients into a blender and incorporate well.

Top with hot water.

This may be a lot for one sitting so you may want to save it and have it later.

You may want to gently warm the mixture on the stovetop to get it warmer.

MAGIC MORNING ELIXIR

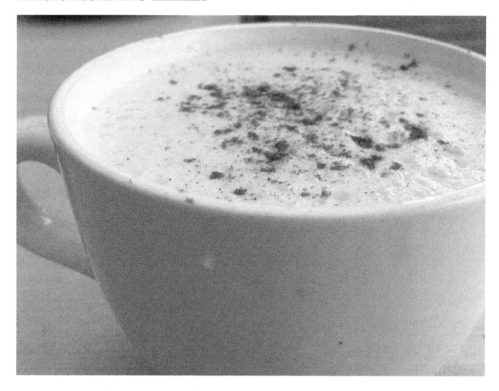

Ingredients:

- 1 tablespoon Dandy Blend (coffee alternative)
- 1 teaspoon Ashwagandha or Maca Powder
- ½ teaspoon cardamom
- 1–2 Tablespoons ghee
- 1–2 Tablespoons unrefined coconut oil
- Hot water (8–16 ounces)
- 2–4 tablespoons full-fat coconut milk
- 5 drops of stevia, or more if you like it sweeter
- Optional: 1 teaspoon Great Lakes unflavored gelatin or psyllium husk powder for a thicker texture.

Directions:

Place all ingredients into a blender and blend until oil emulsifies and elixir thickens.

TENSION TAMER ELIXIR

Ingredients:

- Your favorite stress relief teas, like Yogi Tea's Kava Stress Relief®
- 1 cup hot water
- ¼ cup full-fat coconut milk
- 5 drops of stevia
- 1 drop of vanilla
- 1–2 Tablespoons ghee
- 1–2 Tablespoons unrefined coconut oil
- Optional: 1 teaspoon Great Lakes unflavored gelatin or psyllium husk powder for a thicker texture.

Directions:

Brew your tea base and allow it to steep for 10 minutes.

Strain and set aside.

Combine remaining ingredients with tea in a blender and blend until smooth and drink 1 hour before bed.

Lunch and Dinner

Cauliflower and Greens Stuffed Delicata Squash

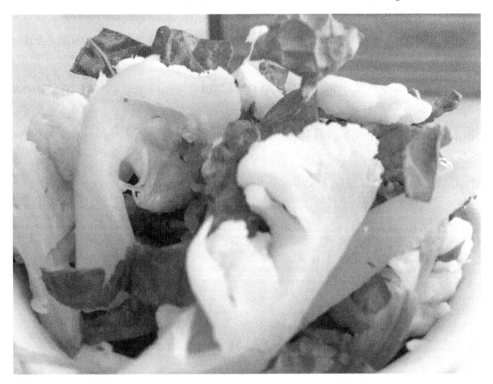

Ingredients:

- 1 delicata squash, cut in half lengthwise, seeds removed
- 1 tablespoon olive oil, ghee, or coconut oil
- 1 clove garlic, minced
- 1 shallot or small onion, thinly sliced
- 5 kale leaves, center vein removed, cut into thin ribbons
- 1 small head of cauliflower, cut into 1-inch pieces
- 1 tablespoon oregano
- Sea salt and pepper to taste

Directions:

Place delicata flesh side down in a Pyrex casserole dish with 1 inch of water and bake for 20–30 minutes at 350.

Meanwhile, in a pot, bring 3 inches of water to a boil and add cauliflower for 5 minutes.

Drain and rinse cauliflower with cold water and then puree in a food processor.

Sauté shallots, garlic and kale until soft and add cauliflower.

Salt to taste.

Stuff this mixture into the baked squash.

GINGER YAM SOUP WITH STEAMED KALE

Ingredients:

- 4 large yams, peeled and cut into 2-inch chunks
- 1 tablespoon ghee
- 1 onion, chopped
- 2 inches peeled fresh ginger
- 1 can regular coconut milk
- ½ cup sunflower seed butter dissolved in ½ cup hot water
- 1 teaspoon lemon juice
- 1 teaspoon cinnamon
- Pinch nutmeg

Directions:

Melt ghee in a soup pot and add onions and ginger.

Sauté for 10 minutes or until onions are soft.

Then place yams in pot with a cup of water and steam until soft.

Add coconut milk and remaining ingredients and bring to a boil and then remove from heat and then blend.

Add salt to taste.

CARROT GINGER SOUP WITH STEAMED KALE

This is a delicious recipe and the addition of the orange gives it a little zip.

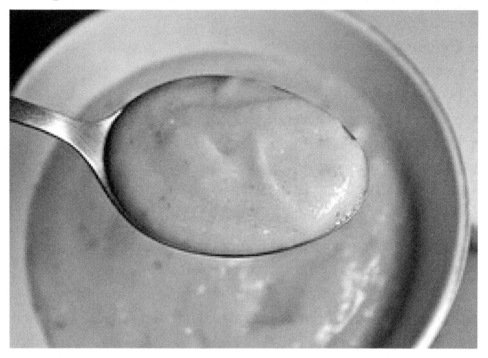

Ingredients:

- 1 yellow onion, diced
- 2 inch piece ginger, peeled and sliced
- 4 stalks celery, sliced
- 6 carrots, sliced
- 2 potatoes, diced
- 1 cup orange juice
- 1 cube Rapunzel vegetable bouillon with herbs
- ½ tablespoon turmeric
- 1 teaspoon dry ginger

Directions:

Place sliced onions in a soup pot on medium high heat and stir occasionally. Adding water if the onions begin to stick.

Add celery, carrots, potatoes, and ginger.

Sauté for about 5 minutes and then add water or veggie stock so that the veggies are covered by about an inch of stock.

Bring to a boil and then turn down heat to a low boil.

Cook until potato is soft.

Then add turmeric, dry ginger, and orange juice.

Remove from heat and blend.

Salt to taste.

BUTTERNUT SQUASH SOUP WITH STEAMED KALE

Ingredients:

- 1 medium-sized butternut squash, peeled, deseeded and cubed
- 1 yellow onion
- 1 inch piece peeled and sliced ginger
- 4 stalks celery, diced
- 2 carrots, diced
- 1 tablespoon Dijon mustard
- 1 splash white wine vinegar
- 2 tablespoons fresh rosemary, minced
- Vegetable stock

Directions:

Sauté onion in a large soup pot until it is tender.

Include the rest of the vegetables, rosemary and sauté for 5 more minutes.

Add veggie stock to cover and bring to a boil.

Cook until squash is tender.

Add Dijon mustard and vinegar.

Turn off heat and serve.

Note about blended soups: *It is not necessary to blend any of the above soups. I like the consistency of a blended soup and they can be used as a sauce for grains like quinoa and basmati rice, but if you like a chunkier stew or don't have a blender that can do the job feel free to not blend them.*

STEAMED KALE

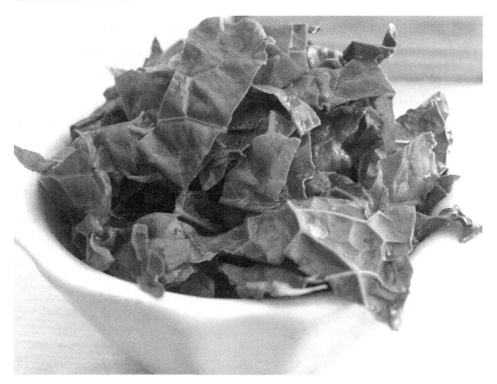

Ingredients:

- 1 bunch of kale, chopped
- 1 splash balsamic vinegar
- 1 tablespoon Italian spice blend
- Optional: toasted sesame seeds

Directions:

Add 2–3 inches of water into a pot and bring to a boil.

Place steam basket in water and add kale.

Cover the pot with a lid, reduce heat, and steam kale for 3–5 minutes.

Remove from heat and toss with vinegar and spices.

Salt to taste.

Oil Massage and Steam

Use the Mahanarayan oil or another food grade oil (sesame, coconut or sunflower) for the *Abhyanga* massage per the instructions provided in the appendix. The skin is considered to be the largest organ in the body and it is continuous with the digestive tract. By nourishing the skin with oil, its natural pharmacy is stimulated and transportation of hormones and vital nutrients to the skin's surface is limited so that these beneficial compounds can support the digestive tract. After an oil massage take a hot shower or sit in a steam room or sauna. The combination of oil and heat allows the pores in the skin to open and receive the oil more fully. Do this at least once a day during the Replacement phase.

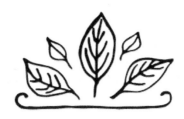

DAY 8 LIQUID DIET

A LIQUID DIET IS NOT EQUIVALENT TO WATER FASTING. IT CONSISTS OF foods that have been liquefied and may be consumed as thick soups, seed-milks, or even food put into the blender with some warm water. Vegetable juices and fruit juices are also okay. The liquid diet can be used up to one time a week under normal circumstances.

Liquid Diet: By having a liquid diet for all three meals on Day 8, you give your body the opportunity to flush out the *ama* that has been loosened by the elixirs and massage during previous days. This procedure does not remove all *ama* from the body, but helps to clean out the major toxins that weaken the digestive forces (*Agni*). This results in a body that will more efficiently digest the Kitchari in the next phase without further *ama* production. At this point, the Kitchari can sustain the body while the detoxifying herbs work to scour the *ama* from the deeper tissues.

Dietary and Beverage Recommendations

- Replace all three meals with a liquid diet.
- Follow the Hydration therapy by sipping warm water every 15 minutes to purify the lymph.
- Drink warm beverages, such as herbal tea, throughout the day.

Lifestyle Recommendations

- Follow the General Home Wellness Guidelines and Daily Guidelines for Healthy Living.

Supplement and Herb Recommendations

- Take 2 Triphala tablets in the evening before bed.
- Take 1 tablet of Sweet Ease and *Kapha/Pitta* Digest before meals.
- Take 1 tablet of Kidney Formula, Immune Support, Turmeric and Shilajit after meals.

Sample Meal Plan for Repair Phase

Day	Breakfast	Lunch	Dinner
Day 8	Nut Milk	West African Bisque	Green Soup

Nut Milks

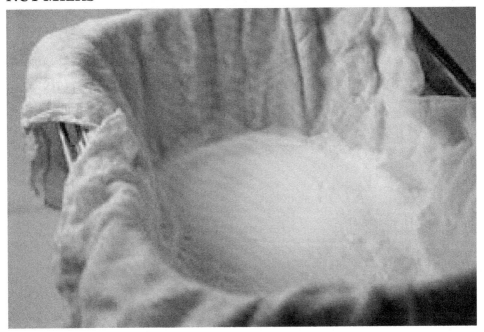

Ingredients:

- 1 cup nuts or seeds, soaked in water for at least 8 hours
- 4 cups water

Directions:

Drain the soaked nuts and discard the soaking liquid.

Blend the nuts or seeds with 4 cups of hot water until the mixture is completely liquefied, smooth, and slightly frothy.

Place cheesecloth or a nut milk bag (use a rubber band to keep them in place) over a jar or bowl (you may also use a fine mesh strainer) and pour the mixture into it.

Squeeze or press the liquid through so that the liquid and nut puree are separated.

Flavor the nut milk with dates, vanilla, cinnamon, etc. based on your preferences.

You can use the leftover nut/seed pulp in morning cereal or as a thickener in soups.

Caution: *Nut/seed milks only keep for several days. Be sure to transfer into an airtight container and keep in the refrigerator.*

WEST AFRICAN CHICKPEA BISQUE

Ingredients:

- 1 yellow onion, diced
- 1 fennel bulb, diced
- 1 tablespoon sesame oil
- 1 medium sweet potato, diced
- 1 cup soaked and cooked chickpeas
- 1 tablespoon lemon juice
- 1 tablespoon grated ginger
- 2 teaspoons chili powder
- 1 teaspoon each: cumin, curry powder, cinnamon
- ¼ cup chopped dates
- 3 tablespoons coconut flour
- ½ bunch of parsley chopped
- ½ cup fresh cilantro

Directions:

Soak chickpeas overnight, drain water and add fresh water to a saucepan, covering the beans by about 2 inches.

Cook until tender about 30–45 minutes. While chickpeas are cooking, sauté onions and fennel in a soup pot until soft, approximately 5 minutes.

Add remaining ingredients (except coconut flour, dates, spices and cilantro) and enough vegetable stock or water to submerge all ingredients.

Bring to a boil and turn down heat so it is at a low boil.

When chickpeas are done, add them to the pot along with enough of their cooking liquid to keep the ingredients submerged.

When the sweet potatoes are tender add spices, seed butter, dates.

Let cool for 10 minutes and then blend ingredients.

Garnish with cilantro.

GREEN SOUP

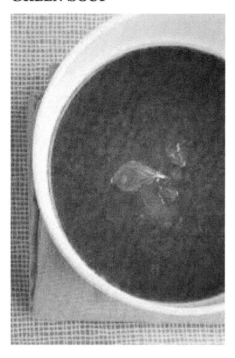

Ingredients:

- 1 cup split peas or whole mung beans
- 1 yellow onion, diced
- 2 stalks of celery, chopped
- 2 zucchini, chopped
- 1 bunch of green leafy vegetables: spinach, chard, kale, arugula, etc.
- 1 bunch of parsley
- 3 cups vegetable stock
- 1 tablespoon Italian seasoning
- 1 tablespoon coriander
- 1 tablespoon curry powder
- Optional
    - Hemp milk and freshly ground flax seed

Directions:

Soak beans in water overnight.

In a large soup pot, sauté onions until tender.

Add the rest of the ingredients, except spinach, and enough water to cover.

Bring to boil and then simmer.

When peas/beans are cooked, remove from heat and add spinach.

Add everything into a blender and blend until smooth.

Add salt and pepper to taste and serve.

For a creamier texture stir a ½ cup of hemp milk with 1 tablespoon of ground flax seed and let sit for 15 minutes. Add this mixture to the soup if you want to thicken it slightly.

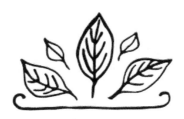

DAY 9–12 REPAIR PHASE

THIS PHASE IS WHAT IS OFTEN CONSIDERED TO BE AN AYURVEDIC cleanse as it employs a cleansing food called Kitchari or mung bean soup. Kitchari is considered to be a complete food and provides optimal nutrition. I have modified the traditional Kitchari recommendations in this procedure to accommodate modern metabolism by creating four options that can be followed. This is the phase when the digestive system is given a break and the appetite is reduced so that the energy and intelligence of the body can be used in order to produce *Ojas*.

Dietary Recommendations

Ayurveda most often relies on a simple porridge-like dish called Kitchari to sustain the body during purification. As the last phase was more rejuvenative this phase has a more detoxifying quality. Kitchari means "mixture," and usually consists of one grain and one bean. Don't worry if you have a hard time digesting the lectins and grains and beans—this will be addressed. It is a nourishing and easy-to-digest meal that works as a simple staple food during the repair phase. The two grains most often used are quinoa and basmati rice but any grain can be used. The beans that are most often used are split mung or green mung dal. When these are mixed with ghee, spices and leafy green vegetables it provides the essential carbohydrates, protein and clean essential fatty acids needed to sustain the body. It is an easy to make one-pot meal that can support the repair of the digestive tract.

Kitchari takes out any confusion or second guessing we may have around what to eat and allows us to avoid all of the questionable foods in our diet known to produce *ama*. In short, Kitchari is *ama*-reducing by virtue of being easy to digest. A Kitchari cleanse is certainly not as radical as a water fast, but it does allow for an extended cleansing time by maintaining basic cellular nutrition. The point is not to prove how long you can go without food, but to give the body enough time away from *ama*-producing foods so that the cleansing herbs and other detoxifying methods can do their work. The deepest cleansing process takes place during this phase. This is when weight loss may occur or when you might find a more beneficial relationship to food. Besides reducing *ama*, you will be cleansed of emotional attachments to unhealthy foods in your life.

As not everyone likes the porridge-like consistency of Kitchari it is recommended to eat it with kraut as well. Not only does this give it a nice crunch in contrast to the porridge, raw fermented vegetables such as kraut are high in probiotics that are beneficial to the gut. As the overall approach is to improve digestive strength, kraut assists in this by assisting the intestinal microbiome.

KITCHARI OPTIONS:

1. Eat Kitchari with kraut.
2. Eat Kitchari and kraut with seasonal vegetable.
3. Eat Kitchari and kraut with fruits, vegetables, beans and grains.
4. Eat Kitchari and kraut with wild game meats or sugar-free protein powder.

When choosing option 3 make sure that your eat fruit separate from other foods. Usually an hour between eating fruit and other foods is plenty.

If you don't tolerate grains and beans then you will want to either choose Option 4 or eat some high quality animal protein with vegetables, or choose Option 3 without the Kitchari. You are not going to create nutrient deficiencies or starve yourself if you don't eat meat for a couple weeks. The most important part is to find a simple meal that will sustain you.

LIFESTYLE RECOMMENDATIONS

- Plan only light work during the Repair phase and only as much exercise as feels appropriate. Yoga is ideal. Light walks or hikes in nature, meditation, and breathing exercises are also ideal during this time.

HERBAL RECOMMENDATIONS

- Continue to take Sweet Ease and *Pitta/Kapha* Digest before meals.
- Increase your intake to 2 tablets of Kidney Formula, Immune System, Turmeric and Shilajit after meals.
  - If you don't tolerate the herbs well, don't increase your dose.

Repair Phase Meal Plan

During the Repair phase we eat Kitchari for three meals a day. If you are trying to lose weight, have low-fat Kitchari (less than 2 teaspoons of oil). If you are finding the Kitchari hard to digest it can be helpful to add more oil. Snacking is not recommended.

Sample Meal Plan for Repair Phase

Day	Breakfast	Lunch	Dinner
Day 1	N/A	Soupy Kitchari	Soupy Kitchari
Day 2	Kitchari with Kraut	Mediterranean Kitchari with kraut	Mexican Kitchari with kraut
Day 3	Kitchari with Kraut	Indian Kitchari with kraut	Thai Kitchari with kraut
Day 4	Kitchari with Kraut	Mediterranean Kitchari with kraut	Mexican Kitchari with kraut
Day 5	Kitchari with Kraut	Indian Kitchari with kraut	Thai Kitchari with kraut

Recipes for the Repair Phase

Like the previous suggestions these recipes can be used as a guide. Feel free to omit or add things to the recipes so that they fit your unique constitution. In general the only rule to follow during this phase is to have Kitchari be the base of your meals, eat 2 tablespoons of kraut with every meal, and to choose one option and stick to it.

A note about Kichari: Some people with small intestinal bacterial overgrowth (SIBO) do not tolerate eating grains and beans. If this is you or if you have a hard time eating grains and beans choose Option 4 and eat wild game meats and veggies with spices instead of Kitchari.

SOUPY KITCHARI

Ingredients:

- 1 cup basmati rice or quinoa
- 1 cup split yellow mung dal
- 6 cups water
- ½ cup water
- ¼ teaspoon salt
- ¼ teaspoon turmeric or mild curry powder
- 1 inch ginger root
- 1 small handful cilantro
- 2 Options: leafy greens
- Optional: 1 tablespoon ghee

Directions:

Soak rice or quinoa and the dahl for 3–8 hours, if you have the time.

In a large saucepan on medium heat, melt ghee and place ginger and turmeric in it.

Stir for a moment until the spices are mixed and fragrant.

Add the remaining ingredients except for leafy greens and water.

Stir until lightly browned or until it starts to stick.

Pour in the 6 cups of water, cover and bring to a boil.

Once it boils, turn down heat to low and cook, lightly covered, until the dahl and rice are soft, about 25–30 minutes.

Add leafy greens at the end.

It will be a soupy consistency.

Basic Kitchari (4 servings)

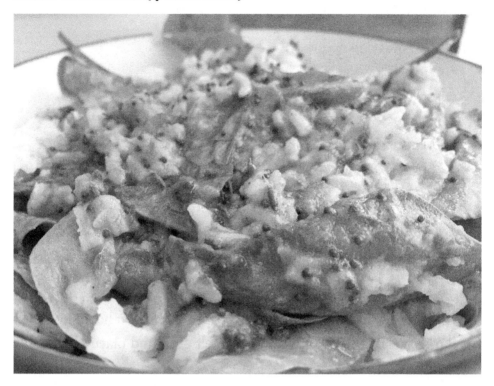

Ingredients:

- ½ cup basmati rice
- 1 cup organic whole or split mung beans. Soaked for at least three hours before cooking.
- 4–6 cups of water
- 2 teaspoons ghee
- 1 teaspoon of black mustard seeds
- 1 teaspoon cumin seeds
- 1 teaspoon fresh grated ginger
- ½ teaspoon of sea salt
- ½ teaspoon of turmeric or mild curry powder
- 1–2 cups chopped vegetables (optional)

Directions:

In a saucepan, warm the ghee.

Add the ginger, mustard seeds, and cumin seeds, then sauté for one to two minutes until the mustard seeds start to pop and the aroma of the spices is released.

Add rice and mung beans and sauté for 2–4 minutes or until they start sticking to the sides of the pot.

Then add 4–6 cups of water, and bring to a boil.

Stir in the turmeric and curry powder, and reduce heat to a simmer.

Cover and cook until beans and rice are tender (about 30–45 minutes) and then add salt.

Your finished Kitchari should be the consistency of a vegetable stew as opposed to a broth.

If you need to add more water, you can.

Taste and add additional salt as needed.

QUINOA KITCHARI

Ingredients:

- 1–½ cups whole green mung beans
- 1 cup quinoa
- 1 burdock root
- 1 parsnip
- 1 bunch broccoli rabe
- 1 sweet potato
- 1 carrot
- 3 stalks celery
- 1 red pepper
- 1 tablespoon turmeric
- 1 teaspoon mustard seeds, fennel seed, cumin seed
- 2 or 3 tablespoons ginger
- ½ tablespoon salt
- 1 cup cilantro
- 1 bunch chard (a little shy of one bunch)

Directions:

Soak beans overnight. Rinse and add 2–½ cups water (you may want to experiment with the amount of water, depending on how soupy you want it). Set aside.

Chop veggies.

Keep ginger and pepper aside.

Heat on medium.

Add ginger and sauté until brown.

Add all seeds.

Add chopped red peppers and sauté for a few minutes before adding turmeric.

Stir in remaining veggies (minus the broccoli, cilantro and chard) for a minute or two.

Add beans that are setting aside in water.

Close lid. Turn heat to high for about 5 or so minutes. Then turn heat to low and cook for another 30 minutes.

Open lid, add broccoli and cook for another 10 minutes.

Turn heat off, mix in chard, cilantro, and salt to taste, close lid and leave for a bit.

Stir in cooked quinoa at the very end.

To cook the quinoa: Add quinoa and 2 cups of water into a saucepan and bring to a boil.

Turn the heat down to low, cover the saucepan, and let simmer for about 15–20 minutes.

When the quinoa looks close to being done, run under cold water until water runs clear.

Keep a little extra water in there, re-heat and cook until perfectly light and fluffy!

Mung Beans	Mudga (Sanskrit)	Vigna radiata

Character: *The Hot Blooded Helper*
Detoxifies the body by supporting the liver and gall bladder and by producing more fluids in the body, which can be used to tonify and lubricate the body. This fluidity can help to relieve *Pitta* in the body. Beans are usually considered diuretic and are used to reduce swelling.

Guna: cool, heavy, dry **Rasa:** sweet, astringent **Vipaka:** sweet **Virya:** cool **Prabhava:** high in protein	**Main Action:** Anti-fever, refrigerant, hemostatic **Action on *Doshas*:** PK-,V+ **Action on *Dhatus*:** Especially good for blood

Description:
As mung beans help to reduce inflammation they can be used in cases of acute food poisoning, dysentery, diarrhea, painful urination, pesticide poisoning, heat stroke, conjunctivitis and edema. In addition to this, skin rashes, thirst, restlessness, impatience and urinary tract infections or other signs of heat can be managed with mung beans. Although less common they have been used in the treatment of high blood pressure, acidosis and ulcers. This is usually due to reducing toxicity in the vascular system.

Externally a paste of mung beans can be used for burns, sores, swelling, inflamed joints, swollen breasts, mastitis.

Main Uses:
Pitta disorders
Convalescence from fever or infectious disease
Detoxes liver from drugs, smoking or alcohol.
Anti-inflammatory and treats cancer, enlarged liver or spleen

Precautions: Do not use when there is excess coldness or deficient digestive fire, such as loose, watery stools and low energy.

SIMPLE KITCHARI

Ingredients:

- 1 cup split yellow mung dal or whole green mung beans
- 1 cup quinoa basmati rice
- 1 tablespoon minced fresh ginger
- 1 tablespoon coconut oil
- 1 teaspoon cinnamon
- ¼ teaspoon cardamom
- ¼ teaspoon clove
- ¼ cup seed milk
- Optional: chia seeds, flax seeds or hemp seeds

Directions:

Soak grains and beans in water. In the morning, drain and rinse grains and beans.

Then place them in a saucepan and fill it with water until it is 1-2 inches above the mixture.

Bring to a boil and add fresh ginger.

Reduce heat and simmer for 20 minutes or until the grains are cooked.

Add remaining ingredients except for seed milk, which will be used to cool off the hot cereal.

MEDITERRANEAN KITCHARI

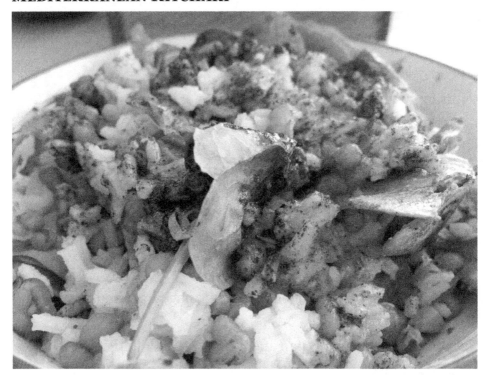

Ingredients:

- 1 cup split yellow mung dal or whole green mung beans
- 1 cup quinoa or basmati rice
- 3 cups water
- 1 leek, diced
- 1 stalk of celery, diced
- 2 carrots, diced
- 1 large tomato, diced
- 1 tablespoon dried basil or 3 tablespoons fresh basil
- 1 teaspoon oregano
- 3 bay leaves
- 1 teaspoon dried rosemary or 1 tablespoon fresh
- ¼ teaspoon black peeper

- 1 tablespoon olive oil
- Optional: garlic, asparagus, spinach, broccoli, peas
- ¼ teaspoon salt

Directions:

Soak grains and beans for 3–8 hours.

In a large saucepan on medium heat, place onion, celery carrots, and bay leaves. Stir frequently for about 5 minutes, adding water so veggies don't stick to the pan.

Then add tomatoes, grains, beans, all spices and water or veggie stock. This is a good time to add optional veggies as well.

Bring to a boil and then let simmer, lightly covered, until grains and beans are cooked (about 20 minutes).

Add olive oil and salt to taste.

MEXICAN KITCHARI

Ingredients:

- 1 cup split yellow mung dal or whole green mung beans
- 1 cup quinoa or basmati rice
- 3 cups water
- 1 onion, diced
- 1 stalk of celery, diced
- 1 handful okra
- 1 bunch of cilantro
- 1 tablespoon oregano
- 1 teaspoon cumin powder
- 1 teaspoon coriander powder
- Optional: garlic, jalapeno, avocado, zucchini, arugula

Directions:

Soak grains and beans for 3–8 hours.

Place the onion, celery, and carrots in a large saucepan on medium-high heat. Stir frequently, adding water so veggies don't stick to the pan and cook for about 5 minutes.

Then add grains, beans, spices, and water or veggie stock (everything except for cilantro). This is a good time to add optional veggies (except for avocado and greens) as well.

Bring to a boil and then let simmer, lightly covered until grains and beans are cooked (about 20 minutes).

Add remaining veggies, cilantro, and salt to taste.

THAI KITCHARI

Ingredients:

- 1 cup split yellow mung dal or whole green mung beans
- 1 cup quinoa or basmati rice
- 3 ½ cups water
- 1 leek, diced
- 1 stalk of celery, diced
- 1 handful shitake mushrooms
- ¼ cup dried coconut
- ¼ cup fresh ginger
- 1 handful of cilantro or Thai basil
- Juice of 1 lime
- Pinch of cayenne pepper
- Salt
- Optional: green beans, bok choy, broccoli, cabbage, asparagus
- 1 tablespoon sesame oil

Directions:

Soak grains and beans for 3–8 hours.

In a large saucepan on medium heat, cook onion, celery and carrots stirring frequently and adding water so veggies don't stick to the pan cooking for about 5 minutes.

In a blender combine ginger, coconut, cilantro or Thai basil, lime juice and ½ cup water and blend until liquefied.

Then add grains, beans, blended items, and water or veggie stock. This is a good time to add optional veggies as well.

Bring to a boil and then let simmer, lightly covered until grains and beans are cooked (about 20 minutes).

Add sesame oil and salt to taste.

Cabbage	Kobi (Hindi)	Brassica oleracea

Character: *The medicinal monk*
Cabbage can be cooked juiced, or fermented. Depending on the way it is prepared, it will have different effects on the body. In general it moistens the intestines, benefits the stomach and improves digestion. This demulcent activity will treat constipation, a dry cough as part of the common cold, mental depression and irritability. Cabbage can also help to removes worms or help heal ulcers.

Guna: cold, light, dry **Rasa:** bitter, pungent **Vipaka:** sweet **Virya:** cool **Prabhava:** Anti-inflammatory	**Main Action:** Alterative, antibacterial, antiviral **Action on *Doshas*:** KP-,V+ **Action on *Dhatus*:** Especially good for blood

Main Uses:
Ulcers and heartburn
Eczema and skin rashes
Infections, or inflammation
Asthma

Cabbage owes its many of its healing properties to its high sulfur content which is why large doses improve circulation warming up cold feet. Cabbage contains iodine and is a rich source of vitamin C and Vitamin A, and Calcium. It is a blood purifier and can help in rashes.

Precautions: Use carefully during nausea and with chronic weakness; it can cause gas when raw.

INDIAN KITCHARI

Ingredients:

- 1 cup split yellow mung dal or whole green mung beans
- 1 cup quinoa or basmati rice
- 1 leek, diced
- 1 stalk of celery, diced
- 1 12-inch burdock root
- 1 tablespoon ghee
- 1 teaspoon black mustard seeds
- 1 teaspoon cumin seeds
- 1 cinnamon stick
- 1 tablespoon fresh minced ginger
- 1 tablespoon turmeric or curry powder
- ¼ teaspoon fenugreek
- Optional: cauliflower, chard, broccoli, green beans, zucchini, peas
- Salt

Directions:

Soak grains and beans for 3–8 hours.

In a large saucepan on medium heat, place cinnamon, mustard seeds and cumin seeds in melted ghee.

Stir for a moment until the spices are mixed and fragrant.

Add remaining spices and onion, celery and carrots, stirring frequently and adding water so veggies don't stick to the pan; cooking for about 5 minutes.

Then add grains, beans, and water or veggie stock. This is a good time to add optional veggies as well.

Bring to a boil and then let simmer, lightly covered, until grains and beans are cooked (about 20 minutes).

Add salt to taste.

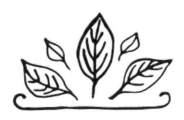

DAY 13–14 POST PHASE

THE LAST COUPLE DAYS ARE A TRANSITION TIME WHERE YOU START TO loosen the reins on what you are required to eat and see what foods from the last 12 days call out to you. The overall approach is to eat simply and to incorporate probiotics and prebiotics into your daily routines.

Dietary Guidelines

As you are nearing the end of the process sometimes it helps to be reminded of why your chose to go through this process and to recommit yourself to your goals. This will help you to consume an appropriate amount of very clean, organic whole foods. An emphasis on steamed vegetables is preferred, though vegetable soups and a light quantity of rice, gluten-free grains, and berries can be included. No junk food or food from a freezer is recommended for at least a week after you have completed program. As a reminder:

- Avoid all meats, processed food, frozen food, yogurt, cheese, ice cream, pizza, honey, and cold drinks for at least a week after the cleanse is complete.
- Don't fast. Eat if you are hungry, don't if you are not. Again, don't overeat.

Include These Recommendations

- Drink 4– 8 ounces of Takra (Indian buttermilk).
- Eat 4 servings of green leafy vegetables.
- Have the gomasio seed mix with every meal.

Lifestyle Guidelines

Observe the following throughout this phase and as you transition into a new routine.

- Avoid strenuous activity. A gentle home yoga practice is perfect.
- Avoid excess exposure to the cold; stay warm, especially the areas of your head and neck.

Herbal Guidelines

The precise way in which you will increase your herbs will vary from person to person depending on their sensitivity to the herbs and the strength of digestion. The overall approach is:

- On Day 13, increase your dose of *Pitta/Kapha* Digest to 2 tablets at every meal.
- If you tolerate this well you can take 3 tablets at every meal on Day 14.
- Then reduce the dosage by one tablet on each consecutive day until you are taking 1 tablet with meals again.
- If you don't tolerate the increase of the herbs well. Then take a larger dose at lunch and only 1 tablet at breakfast and dinner.

Sample Meal Plan for Post Phase

Day	Breakfast	Snack	Lunch	Snack	Dinner
Day 13	Yam Breakfast Pudding with coconut yogurt	Takra	Red Lentil Dahl with gomasio	Takra	Thai Coconut Soup with gomasio
Day 14	Poached apples and berries with strawberry sunflower cream	Takra	Thai Coconut Soup with gomasio	Takra	Red Lentil Dahl with gomasio

Recipes for the Post-Cleanse

SWEET TAKRA

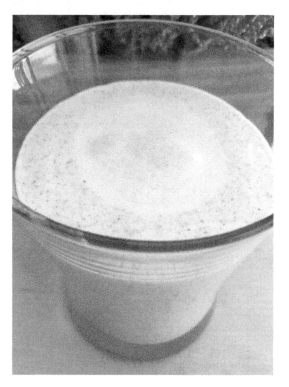

Ingredients:

- ½ cup Nancy's whole milk yogurt or greek yogurt
  - Note: If you don't tolerate yogurt well, use coconut yogurt recipe below.
- ½ cup water
- 1 teaspoon cinnamon
- 1 teaspoon cardamom
- 1 teaspoon fennel powder

Directions:

Mix spices into yogurt. Then mix water into yogurt mix.

Savory Takra

Ingredients:

- ½ cup Nancy's whole milk yogurt or greek yogurt
  - **Note:** *If you don't tolerate yogurt well, use coconut yogurt recipe below.*
- ½ cup water
- 1 teaspoon cumin
- 1 teaspoon coriander
- 1 teaspoon fennel powder
- Pinch of salt

Directions:

Mix spices into yogurt. Then mix water into yogurt mix.

GOMASIO SEED POWDER

Ingredients:

- 2 tablespoons chia seeds
- 2 tablespoons flaxseeds
- 2 tablespoons sesame seeds
- 1 teaspoon. cumin seed
- 1 teaspoon coriander seed
- 1 teaspoon fennel seed
- 2 tablespoons licorice powder
- 1 teaspoon sea salt

Directions:

Place all ingredients into a spice grinder and grind into a fine powder. You can double or triple the proportions so that you have 1 teaspoon on hand to be added to your food.

Most ingredients can be found in the bulk department at your nearest health food store.

BREAKFASTS

YAM BREAKFAST PUDDING

Ingredients:

- ½ cup baked winter squash or sweet potato
- 1 tablespoon ground flaxseeds
- ½ teaspoon. cinnamon
- Pinch sea salt
- 8–10 drops liquid stevia or dash of raw honey
- 1 teaspoon. coconut oil

Directions:

Combine all ingredients in a food processor and process until smooth. Serve.

COCONUT YOGURT

Ingredients:

- 1 can full-fat Native Forest coconut milk
- 3 capsules of probiotics (my favorite brand is GutPro)

Directions:

Place the contents of the probiotic capsule into the coconut milk and let ferment for 24–48 hours in a glass jar with a plastic lid closed loosely. Then place the yogurt in the fridge and use it for your takra.

POACHED APPLES AND BERRIES WITH STRAWBERRY SUNFLOWER CREAM

Ingredients:

- 1 Fuji apple
- 1 pint of blueberries

Directions:

Bring water to a boil and place sliced Fuji apples in the water for 1 minute and then place the blueberries into the water and cook for an additional minute.

Then strain and cover with sunflower cream.

STRAWBERRY SUNFLOWER CREAM

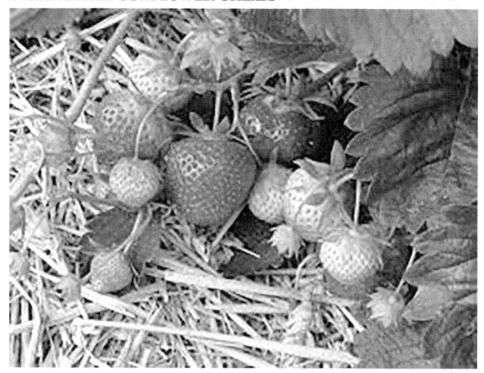

Ingredients:

- 1 cup soaked sunflower seeds
- 1–2 dates
- ½ cup of strawberries
- 1 teaspoon cinnamon
- 1 teaspoon cardamom
- 1 splash of vanilla

Directions:

Blend all ingredients in a food processor.

Lunch and Dinner
Red Lentil Dahl

Ingredients:

- 1 tablespoon coconut oil
- 2 cloves of garlic (or 1 teaspoon. minced)
- 1 small/medium onion, chopped
- 1 cup red lentils
- 1–2 tablespoons Madras curry powder
- ½ teaspoon sea salt
- 3 cups water
- 1 cup tomatoes, chopped
- ¼ cup full-fat coconut milk
- ½ lemon, juiced

Directions:

Heat coconut oil on medium heat in a soup pot and sauté garlic and onion until soft.

Add lentils, curry powder, and salt.

Add water and cook 30–40 minutes until lentils are soft.

Add tomatoes and cook another 5–10 minutes.

Stir in coconut milk and lemon juice.

Add salt to taste.

Thai Coconut Vegetable Soup

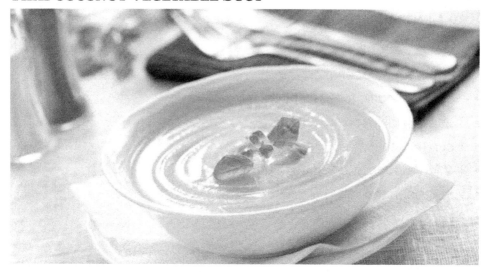

Ingredients:

- 1 shallot, cut into half moons
- 2 cups sliced shiitake mushrooms
- 3 carrots, julienned
- 1 (13.5-oz.) can full-fat coconut milk
- 3 cups vegetable broth
- 2 zucchini, cut in half lengthwise and sliced
- 2 cups bok choy, sliced (chop greens)
- ½ cup chopped cilantro
- 1 tablespoon wheat-free tamari or sea salt to taste
- Optional: Juice of 1 lime

Directions:

Sauté shallots and mushrooms on medium high heat in a soup pot, adding water so that it doesn't stick.

After 10 minutes, add carrots, coconut milk and broth and bring to boil.

Then lower heat to simmer and then add bok choy, cilantro, and salt.

COMPLETION OF THE RE-SOLUTION PROGRAM

YOU WILL KNOW WHEN THE PROGRAM IS COMPLETE WHEN YOU EXPERI-
ence the following (or an improvement in these areas):

- Regular bowel movements
- No gas
- Clean tongue (very little coating)
- Fresh breath
- No lethargy or heaviness in the body and mind
- Lightness in the body with good energy
- A general sense of happiness

You may find that afterwards you will enjoy eating light for some time. An occasional day in which you eat only Kitchari is suggested in the weeks following the program. Should you feel an impulse to indulge in questionable foods, eating light can serve to further break the link with that food. After you have broken the link, start slowly introducing more complex foods.

Most importantly, Ayurveda recognizes that each person is uniquely different. Follow your own body's wisdom; listen to its requests. Do your best, however, to know the difference between a true bodily need and an impulse for something habituated to the mind.

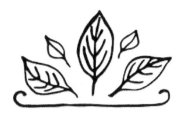

WHAT TO DO AFTER THE POST PHASE

Elimination Test Diet

Samsarajana Krama means a graduated diet and often refers to an incremental increase in the consumption of food after a purge. In this context we are using the principles of *Samsarjana Krama* to test for food allergies. Since many allergies and sensitivities cannot be clearly identified using blood or skin tests, this has been found to be an un-invasive ways to help identify the foods that may be causing physical and or behavioral symptoms. Blood tests often test for antibodies and many patients report that they have high antibodies to the foods that they eat the most of. Many patients do not have symptoms in response to these foods even though the blood test shows that they are producing antibodies to these foods. Skin allergy tests are relatively invasive, as they require puncturing the skin in order to expose the blood to a possible allergen.

Samsarjana Krama is utilized after a prolonged period (2 to 4 weeks) on an elimination diet. During this time, common food allergens are eliminated completely. Examples of these include: gluten, dairy, sugar, soy, caffeine, nuts, corn, alcohol, citrus, sulfites, condiments, food additives and eggs. *Samsarjana Krama* is considered the challenge period where the foods that have been eliminated are added in gradually.

How it Works:

1. Eliminate common food allergens for 2–4 weeks.
2. Pick one challenging food to introduce and introduce it for 3 days in a row, keeping a detailed record of reactions. During this time, make sure not to introduce any other food allergens.
3. If significant symptoms do occur, stop eating the challenge food immediately, record reaction and resume the elimination diet for at least 24 symptom-free hours before choosing your next challenge food.
4. Schedule an appointment to discuss the results of *Samsarjana Krama*.

Each of us is curious about different foods and you may not want to challenge all the foods that you have eliminated at one time. Thus the food that you choose to challenge first may be different than someone else. Below is an example of how to perform *Samsarjana Krama*. The approach and sequence can be used as a model for your own testing.

How to Challenge:

These are only suggestions and recommendations of foods and quantities to use. You want to make sure to eat enough to stimulate a reaction if one is possible, but not so much that you feel terrible if you do get a reaction. On Days 2 and 3, resume the elimination diet and pay close attention to how your body responds to the challenge food that was consumed on Day 1. Day 4 is a buffer and then you can resume challenging with a different food on Day 5. For example:

Day 1: Dairy

- Use 1 cup of cow's milk on elimination-friendly cereal for breakfast
- Have 1–2 ounces of hard cheese with lunch
- Make a cream sauce for elimination-friendly pasta

Day 2: Observe and record

Day 3: Observe and record

Day 4: Buffer

Day 5: Eggs

- Have a poached or basted egg for breakfast
- Have a hardboiled egg on a salad for lunch
- Have scrambled eggs with dinner

Day 6: Observe and record

Day 7: Observe and record

Day 8: Buffer

Day 9 Gluten: *(Note: Use a non-wheat gluten source.)*

- 1 cup cooked oatmeal for breakfast
- Sandwich with 100% rye bread for lunch
- Barley soup for dinner

Day 10: Observe and record

Day 11: Observe and record

Day 12: Buffer

Day 13: Wheat: *(Note: Use 100% whole wheat.)*
- Shredded wheat with rice milk for breakfast
- Wheat bread sandwich for lunch
- 1 cup pure wheat pasta for dinner

Day 14: Observe and record

Day 15: Observe and record

Day 16: Buffer

Day 17: Soy:
- 1 cup soymilk with elimination friendly cereal
- 1 cup baked tofu with lunch
- 1 cup edamame with dinner

Continue this series until you have challenged each of the foods you wish.

If you have very severe symptoms *and a strong reaction, it is best to call 911. This is very rare, but it is not worth risking anaphylaxis. Symptoms can vary widely by individual. Common symptoms to food allergens include gas, bloating, fatigue, diarrhea, nausea, rashes, dry skin, runny nose, congestion, cramps, and bad breath. More rare symptoms include joint pain, difficulty remembering, and difficulty sleeping, itching, and sweating.*

REJUVENATION FROM THE INSIDE OUT

REJUVENATION IS AN AYURVEDIC PRACTICE THAT IS USED TO REPLENISH the vital energy of the body from a cellular level. It is most often done after a cleanse, when the body and mind are feeling light. Removing toxicity from the system allows us to improve the cellular nutrition and re-invigorate the intelligence of the body from the ground up. In this way, rejuvenation ultimately is the aim of cleansing. A cleanse is like bleaching a piece of fabric and rejuvenation is dying the fabric with the colors and designs that are going to support our long-term health.

What's an Appropriate Period of Time?

While more is usually better when it comes to rejuvenation, a general recommendation is to perform rejuvenation for an amount of time equal to the duration of your cleanse. For example if you just completed a two-week cleanse then you would want to do rejuvenation for 14 days. Most people really enjoy rejuvenation as it is very nourishing to the body, emotions, and mind.

Dietary Rejuvenatives

After a cleanse it is very important not to overwhelm digestion. Choose from the foods below, but remember that these are high quality foods and do not need to be taken in high quantity.

Nuts and Seeds: Choose nuts and seeds from the below list. A ½ cup of soaked nuts or seeds a day is the best way to rejuvenate the tissues. You can soak the nuts for eight hours with sea salt for extra flavor and put them in a toaster oven on low heat for 20–30 minutes to make them more crunchy.

- Almonds
- Cashews
- Brazil nuts
- Sesame seeds
- Coconut
- Hemp seeds

Fruits: Fruits are best taken alone or with other carbohydrates like grains or vegetables. Eat less than 2 tablespoons of fat or protein if included with fruits. The fruits below build the blood and the vital fluids.

- **Wild fruits:** huckleberry, juneberry, hawthorn, thimbleberry
- **Cultivated berries:** strawberry, raspberry, cranberry, etc.
- **Stone fruits:** apricot, plum peach, cherry
- **Stewed dried fruit:** dates, raisins, and gogi berries

Grains: Support the body and mind by bringing a feeling of satisfaction and fullness. They are great for rejuvenation, but like everything else diversity and moderation are key. In order to improve vitality, choose non-grass cereal grains.

- Teff
- Amaranth
- Kamut
- Wild rice
- Buckwheat
- Millet

- Oat
- Barley

Dairy: In nationalities that tolerate dairy well, dairy can be a great addition to a rejuvenation program as it nourishes the entire body by a very precise blend of fat, sugar, and protein. ½–1 cup of warm milk with a pinch of cardamom 3–5 times a week as a snack or meal replacement can be a great addition to rejuvenation.

- Raw goat and cow milk or heavy cream
- Hemp milk
- Almond milk
- Hazelnut milk

Meat: The nutrient density in meat makes it remarkable for nourishing the body. As it is higher on the food chain it also has a high concentrations to chemicals that are accumulated from the air, soil, and water. For this reason, it is best to eat meat 3–5 times a week or less. The best meat sources are wild game meats but free-range organic meat is also fine. Making a stock with the bones of these animals is the best way to receive the nutrition from meat without compromising digestion.

- **Wild game meats:** venison, elk, caribou and moose
- **Wild cold water fish:** salmon, pike, char, sardines, smelt, herring
- **Pasture raised poultry:** chicken, duck, turkey and pheasant
- **Free range meats:** lamb, goat, bison and mutton

Spices: The foods that provide the most benefit for rejuvenation are nutrient dense foods that are fully digested. Spices can help in this regard by facilitating the conversion of this dense nutrition into bioavailable nutrients for the body. Choose spices that are warming and slightly sweet to improve digestion.

- **Three C's:** cumin, coriander, and cardamom
- Saffron, ginger, and vanilla
- Oregano, citrus, and fennel
- Allspice, cinnamon, and nutmeg
- Curry powder, turmeric, and fenugreek

Oils: Oils are a remarkable food and a testament to the energy that goes into their extraction. Because of this complicated process, oils are also relatively fragile and can degrade when exposed to heat. The most fragile oils are walnut, hemp, borage, and fish oils. These oils oxidize swiftly and should not be consumed unless you are making them yourself. Other options are:

- Extra virgin sesame oil: low-medium heat, 350F/175C
- Extra virgin coconut oil (not copra): low medium heat, 350F/175C
- Extra virgin olive oil: medium heat 405F/210C
- Extra virgin almond oil: medium heat, 420F/216C
- Organic palm and palm kernel oil: medium heat, 455F/235C
- Organic grass-fed ghee: high heat: 485F/252C
- Extra virgin avocado oil: high heat, 520F/271C

Rejuvenative Herbs: The synergy that is able to happen in an herbal formula usually exceeds the benefits that can be derived from taking a singular herb. Rejuvenative herbs are tonifying, adaptogenic, and building for the entire system. Choose a formula that includes some of the following herbs:

- **Ashwagandha** — adaptogen, anti-inflammatory, antioxidant, immune amphoteric, antitumor, nervine, antispasmodic, mild astringent, diuretic.
- **Shatavari** — adaptogen, antibacterial, antispasmodic, aphrodisiac, demulcent, diuretic, immune tonic, lung tonic, galactagogue, gastroprotective.
- **Amalaki** — adaptogen, anti-inflammatory, antioxidant, antiviral, laxative, diuretic, lowers cholesterol.
- **Schizandra** — adaptogen, antioxidant, anti-inflammatory, immune tonic, astringent, hepatoprotective, nervine, expectorant.
- **Tulsi** — adaptogen, antibacterial, antidepressant, antioxidant, antiviral, carminative, diuretic, expectorant, galactagogue, immunomodulator.
- **Astragulus** — adaptogen, antibacterial, antioxidant, antiperspirant, heart tonic, hepatoprotective, immune tonic.
- **Guduchi** — adaptogen, anti-inflammatory, antioxidant, cholinergic, diuretic, febrifuge, hepatoprotective, immune amphoteric.
- **Licorice** — adaptogen, antiviral, antidiuretic, antihistamine, anti-inflammatory, antioxidant, antitumor, demulcent, expectorant, hepatoprotective, immunomodulator.

Rejuvenative Lifestyle: Rejuvenation is similar to cleansing in that it requires us to slow down so that we can use our energy for self-repair and internal activities instead of using all of our energy to accomplish external tasks. Some routines that can be beneficial during rejuvenation are:
- Daily Abhyanga
- Slow down, rest more
- Less time on computers
- Gentle exercise

Cultivating vitality and internal strength allows us to refill our tank so that we can make the journey of our life with ease. Taking time now to do rejuvenation will make us more resilient toward disease. Consider following this year's cleanse with some more nutrient dense foods, healing herbs, and a couple more weeks of slowing down.

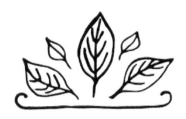

COMMON EXPERIENCES AND BODILY SENSATIONS

The results of cleansing is different for every person and with every different kind of cleanse. Although you may experience some challenges, cultivate determination and remember that the feeling on the other side is well worth your efforts.

Common Experiences

- Mild fatigue
- Anger
- Frustration with yourself
- Frustration with your partner
- Frustration with your kids
- Weight loss
- A sense of relief
- Clearer skin
- Better elimination
- Freedom from deciding what to eat
- Elimination of cravings
- Lack of or decreased appetite
- Brighter eyes
- A stronger body odor
- Skin breakouts
- Mild headaches from caffeine withdrawal

- Resistance to doing this, even though you've made the commitment to yourself
- Feelings of justification for wanting to quit
- Sadness
- Balance, calm, clarity

Everyone responds differently to cleansing. Some feel euphoric and some struggle; most feel a little of both. Everyone will experience some mild discomfort or withdrawal from a food or habituated substance and finish with a more vibrant and clear body and mind.

Everyone has a different phase that challenges them and, since we are all unique, the sensations and challenges at each stage will be different for each person. Below is a list of possible experiences:

- This process may bring an unexpected increase in *Vata Dosha* and its qualities, such as anxiety, nervousness, dryness and coldness, lightheadedness, and an ungrounded and impulsive desire (cravings) for comfort foods (sweets, salty foods or just familiar foods from childhood). In most cases, these sensations arise from a true *Vata* aggravation, meaning that the body is lightening too quickly and the Space (*akash*) and Air (*vayu*) elements are increasing too rapidly. This is to be expected and should be tolerated to a point. Should it occur, modestly increase the amount of food you consume until the sensation goes away. By the second or third day, you should begin to experience more energy and feel lighter in your body. That is a sign that the body is cleansing and beginning to function more optimally without aggravating *Vata*. You may still feel some of these *Vata* signs, but they should pass within a few days.
- You may also feel a sensation of warmth. That is the body working to access its reserves of energy in the layers of body fat. The

process is known as thermogenesis, in which the metabolic rate increases, burning fat to release heat as energy—this is good for weight loss. It's not unusual to lose 10 pounds or more during the two weeks.

- In some cases, especially in those with eating disorders (most of us have an eating disorder to some degree), the associated *samskara* (engrained karmic habit) that reinforces the eating disorder may struggle with the emerging discipline-based freedom that this process cultivates. If and when the *samskara* reemerges (and it will) *chitta* (discrimination) concedes to the more powerful *samskara*. In plain speak, we spiritually "fall asleep" and, in the unconscious state, we give in to our weakness. This struggle will play itself out most intensely within the first few days of the cleanse and in the few weeks afterwards. It is suggested that you stay alert to this dynamic and devote yourself to the power (*Shakti*) of a conscious mind and heart.

Solutions to Common Discomforts

Like all common experiences, the discomforts that come into our lives are opportunities to tune in and make deeper connections to your body's connection to food.

CONSTIPATION

The myriad of complex factors that can be responsible for infrequent bowel movements are many and it takes investigating the patterns of your life and routines to truly get to the bottom of things, but a combination of these suggestions will help:

- If you're doing too much while you're cleansing, it could make your body hold on to excess to try and nourish itself. First, reduce your schedule and spend more time relaxing.

- Increase your dosage of Triphala to up to 8 tablets before bed.
- At night, boil 1 tablespoon of flax seed in 1 cup of water for 2–3 minutes and drink the entire mixture.
- Drink prune juice until the bowels normalize. About a ½ cup a day.
- For more severe constipation, give yourself an enema. Make Triphala tea by steeping 1 teaspoon of Triphala powder in 1 cup of hot water. After the tea has returned to just below body temperature (lukewarm), use the tea in an enema.
- You may want to increase the amount of fat that you are eating as that can help lubricate the bowels.
- Supplements that can be used to aid elimination are probiotics by GutPro or Magnesium in the form of CALM. You can also drink a ¼ cup of aloe vera juice to help.
- Make sure you are drinking enough water.
- Look at your intentions and focus your mind on tuning in to your release and Re-solution and celebrate that it doesn't have to be so hard
- Consider doing simple twisting poses (seated, standing or on your back). No need to be a yoga pro, just lay on your back and let your knees drop to one side and hold for a minute or so while taking nice deep belly breaths. Squatting can also help get the downward energy moving, so if that's accessible in your body, you can do a low squat with your feet turned out and butt dropped low (and think about releasing).

Sleep Disturbances

- When your sleep is disturbed it is important to determine whether there is anything else different than usual. This could be foods that may be stimulating, an increase in your stress levels, or a change in your normal bedtime.

- Sometimes the program can give you more energy than you are ready for. Increasing the amount of fat in your diet, especially before bed will help you ground. Consider drinking heated coconut or almond milk with nutmeg before bed.

Itchy Skin

Sometimes bumps, swelling or itchy skin can result as part of a detox reaction. By improving the function of the gut you can help your skin. This includes warm baths, more fat, and increasing your omega 3's with the gomasio seed powder. Avoid putting things on the skin as that can clog the pores and stop things from trying to move out.

Neck Pain

Achiness and pain can be part of the detox reaction and it can be helpful to receive some lymph massage, baths, soaking your feet, and castor oil packs. It can also be useful to vent either in a journal to a trusted friend or elsewhere.

Feeling full but not satisfied

If you are eating enough to be full, but not being satisfied it may be an indication that you are need of some extra self-nurturing, perhaps an Epsom salt bath. Whatever it is that helps you feel your best.

ITCHING AND SWELLING

If it is an allergic reaction, then look for new things that you have added to your diet or your protocol. The inclusion of fermented foods can sometimes lead to die-off reactions that appear through the skin. Make sure that you don't get depleted. Consider soaking your feet with Epsom salts.

SEVERE FATIGUE OR LETHARGY

Sometimes removing gluten, dairy, sugar and coffee all at once can lead to a detox reaction that includes fatigue. Honing in on it may take some time, so in the meantime I would consider doing the following:

- Take an Epsom salt bath with 2 cups of salt once a day.
- Do a castor oil pack before bed.
- Make sure you are drinking plenty of water.
- Use the above recommendations for constipation as well.

DARK CIRCLES UNDER THE EYES

This can be an indication of a food allergy, a lack of sleep, or poor quality sleep. Dietary strategies can be used to increase the amount of good fats you are eating and include vitamins like E and A.

BLOATING

When it comes to bloating and gas, it can be helpful to look back at your elimination for the past days. Sometimes loose stools can draw water out of the colon. Beans may also be the culprits, in which case it may be time to take a break from them.

Gas

Gas can come from an increase in fiber and eating too much food.

Anxiety

This usually arises because your feel anxious about your food. By making more time in your schedule to prepare food, and taking time before eating to take a few breaths while you visualize your body breaking down the food, you can help alleviate anxiety. You can also make sure you are getting enough green leafy vegetables to increase your B vitamins and make sure that you are getting enough good fats. You may also need to be eating more protein in the form of beans and nuts.

Headaches

In the beginning you may get mild headaches as your body lets go of old habits. If this happens, here are some suggestions:
- Drink plenty water to stay hydrated.
- Place a cool ice cloth on the forehead and put heat on the feet for 20–30 minutes, until the headache subsides.
- Use peppermint essential oil on the temples.

Sinus Congestion

If your sinuses are feeling congested from all the fat, then you may want to consider using a neti pot and Nasya oil. In order to do Neti, start with a cleaned and disinfected neti pot (I use a porcelain neti pot and clean it with hot water and soap after every use). Fill it with warm (not too hot!) water and about ¼ teaspoon of salt, if it tastes like tears it is usually the right amount. Angle and bend the head slightly to the side so the water pours into the nostril that is higher than other one that the fluid is running out of. Breathe through your mouth and allow the water to gently flow in one nostril and out the other passively. When complete you can let the nostril drain and then do the other side. DO NOT BLOW YOUR NOSE! You can swallow any mucus down the back of your throat and spit it out, but at no time should you blow out of your nostrils. When this is complete, do Nasya oil by placing three to five drops of medicated oil into your nostril. You can also use your pinky finger to apply this.

Low Blood Sugar

If you are finding yourself fatigued or consistently famished, it may be that your blood sugar is low. Add lean protein like turkey or bone broth to your lunch and see if that helps. You can also use a nonfat protein powder, such as whey, rice or vegetable protein powder if needed.

APPENDIX I

General Recommendations For Balance

To Balance Heaviness	To Balance Intensity	To Balance Over-activity
Be Active	*Be Calm*	*Be Moderate*
Stimulating activities	Rest and relax	Adequate sleep
Physical labor	Cut down schedule	Avoid late nights
Stay warm, stay active	Cut down striving	Disciplined schedule
Sunbathing	Stay cool	Regular hours
Less sleep (shorter nights rest, no naps)	Take in cool breezes	Sexual moderation
Mix it up (variety of activities)	Gardens and gardening, flowers	Mild physical effort
Avoid cold and damp	Contentment	Avoid wind and cold
Cultivate physical challenges	Forgiveness	Avoid overwork
Mental stimulation	Simplify your life	Avoid all types of stress
Promote travel	Avoid the sun	Avoid intense travel
Avoid "couch potato" behavior	Take in moonlight	Avoid excess stimulation (TV, etc.)

Life Force Enhancing Exercises

- Walk barefoot on the earth for 10 minutes every day. Intend to absorb nourishment from Mother Earth.
- Walk along natural bodies of water. Allow cooling, coherent influence of water to infuse you.
- Allow light and warmth of sun to permeate you.
- Take a walk where there is abundant vegetation and deeply inhale the breath of the plants.
- Gaze into the heavens at night. Let your awareness touch the stars and the furthest reaches of the cosmos.

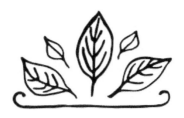

APPENDIX II

Abhyanga: Ayurvedic Daily Self Oil Massage

> *"The body of one who uses oil massage regularly is not affected much even if subjected to accidental injuries or strenuous work. By using oil massage daily, a person is endowed with pleasant touch, trimmed body parts and becomes strong, charming and least affected by old age."*
>
> —*Charaka Samhita*

Abhyanga is the anointing of the body with oil. Often medicated and usually warm, the oil is massaged into the entire body before bathing. It can be beneficial for maintaining health and used as a medicine for certain disorders. Abhyanga can be incorporated into a routine appropriate for almost everyone.

The Sanskrit word *sneha* means both "oil" and "love," and the effects of Abhyanga are similar to the effect of saturation with love. Both experiences can give a deep feeling of stability, warmth and comfort. Sneha is *sukshma*, or "subtle." This Subtlety allows the oil to pass through minute channels in the body and penetrate deep layers of tissue.

Ayurveda teaches us that there are seven *dhatus*, or layers of tissue in the body. Each layer is successively more concentrated and life giving. It is taught that for the effects of *sneha* to reach to the deepest layer, the oil should be massaged into the body for 800 *matras*, roughly five minutes. If we consider that the entire body needs this kind of attention, a 15-minute massage is the minimum amount of time for Abhyanga.

Sneha (oil) used on the human organism imparts a tone and vigor to its tissues in the same manner that water furnishes the necessary nutritive elements to the roots of a tree or a plant, when poured into the soil it fosters growth. The use of *sneha* at a bath causes the *sneha* to penetrate into the system through the mouths of the veins (*siras*) and the ducts (*dhamanis*) of the body, as also through the roots of the hair, and thus soothes and invigorates the body with its own essence.

PROCEDURE

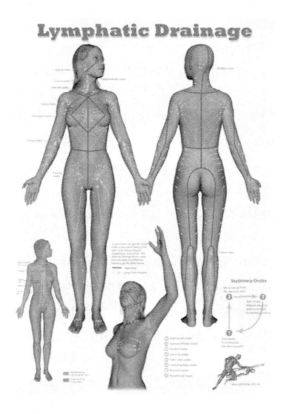

Use Mahanarayan oil or sesame oil. If neither one is suitable you may also try olive oil or coconut oil. The oil should be heated slightly above body temperature. Ideally, about 10–20 minutes should be spent each morning on the massage. If you don't have time, however, it is better to do a very brief massage than to skip it altogether. In general, use circular strokes on the joints and long strokes on the limbs, massaging toward your heart. Move everything back towards the heart using the lymphatic drainage picture to the left as a guide.

Head massage: Start by massaging the head. Place a small amount of oil on the fingertips and palms and begin to massage the scalp vigorously. Then move onto the forehead, cheekbones, chin, nose, and around the eyes. Hold tender areas and breath.

Face and ears: Apply oil gently with the open part of the hand to your face and outer part of your ears.

Neck: Massage the front and back of your neck, and the upper part of your spine. Continue to use your open hand in a rubbing type of motion.

Body application: Apply a small amount of oil to your entire body and then proceed with the massage to each area of the body.

Arms, hands and fingers: Next massage your arms. The proper motion is back and forth, over your long bones, and circular over your joints. Massage both arms, including hands and fingers.

Chest and abdomen: Apply oil to the chest and abdomen. A very gentle circular motion should be used over your heart. Over the abdomen, follow the bowel pattern moving from right to left.

Back and spine: Massage the back and spine. There will be some area that you may have difficulty reaching, just do the best you can.

Legs and feet: Massage the legs, like the arms, use a back and forth motion over the long bones and circular over the joints. Massage the bottoms of the feet. The feet are considered especially important because they relate to the rest of the body. Use the open part of the hand and massage vigorously back and forth over the soles of the feet.

Release Depleting Emotions, Cultivate Love

All of us have experienced pain and disappointment in the past. This is part of life. When we are restricted by these experiences in the present we lose our ability to live fully. By understanding how your emotional reaction to a person or situation creates your interpretation, you can then determine your response to a situation. When you are feeling emotional, take a moment to answer these questions:

- What is your heart telling you?
- How do you feel about the occurrence?

EMOTIONS AND AYURVEDA

How a situation affects you depends on your emotional reaction and your internal conversation, not on the external situation itself. When we become conscious of these elements it gives us a different or better way of interpreting a situation. Our internal landscape can be changed and we can choose how we perceive and interpret situations and hopefully loosen our habitual patterns of using a limited, unproductive viewpoint and shift our focus. Each of us has beneficial patterns that can be illuminated by the *Doshas*:

- *Kapha*s cherish stability and consistency in thought, word and deed; they are challenged by change and dynamism. When there is too much change in their lives they feel hurt. Focus on *Kapha*'s impulse to look beyond diversity and find common ground.
- *Pitta*s are challenged by qualities that are not in control, unconcerned with power, and lighthearted and carefree. In order to stay in control *Pitta* reacts to stress with anger. Concentrate on *Pitta*'s drive to discern in order to see the truth of your reaction to the situation.
- *Vata*s are challenged by discipline, loyalty and consistency. When *Vata* types are able to encourage routine in their lives it helps their dominant emotion of fear. Embody *Vata*'s tendency to change their approach and their minds in order to start new routines and rituals.

By aligning with our natural tendency we recognize our true nature, access our quiet inner voice of wisdom, and relinquish any need to be right or defend. This allows us to become more conscious of our choices and stop judgments and defensiveness used to create our boundaries.

FIVE KEYS TO EMOTIONAL BOUNDARIES
I am responsible for my emotional life.
Without knowing it, most of us have established a pattern of predictable emotional reactions based on our past conditioning. Hurt, anger, sadness, and fear are authentic emotions that will occur as long as we are alive. These emotions are natural indicators that our personal boundaries have been crossed. Explore the behaviors and activities that place you in a situation that recurrently leads to an unwelcome crossing of your boundaries and a wounded feeling.

You have a choice about engaging in these activities. A more core choice is allowing hurtful words to consistently trigger you. Learn to not take things personally. Place someone's rude behavior in a context. It is impossible to know the pain and hurt that creates their behavior. As you are responsible for your reaction to the situation, take a deep breath and respond openly and honestly in order to fully process the experience so that you don't carry it with you.

I set emotional boundaries with a balance of strength and flexibility.

We may over- or under-respond to our emotional boundaries being crossed and become upset or angry, lash out, accuse, deny, withdraw, become sarcastic, or mope. The purpose of these reactions is to re-establish a boundary that allows us to feel safe and in control of our own lives. Your reactions reflect the best emotional response you are capable of. Does your emotional response maintain your boundary without overreacting? If not, how can you expand your choices to improve your sense of safety? Does your response expend sufficient energy to restore the boundary without creating unnecessary repercussions?

Setting clear boundaries and responding proportionately to trespasses are the secrets to emotional health. Pay close attention to any experience that triggers your alarm system to go into overdrive. Over-compensation is the primary cause of losing energy and leads to emotional nosedives. With careful attention you will be able to keep your interpretations of situations from making mountains out of molehills.

I favor emotional exchanges based on equality and avoid exchanges that foster power imbalances.

When an emotional exchange is based on equality it is energizing to both parties because it is based on mutual acceptance and authenticity. When we accept others as they are, we create vibrant relationships. When a relationship is based on power discrepancies, a struggle between both parties to maintain control can be depleting. We are responsible for our words and actions and we cannot take vitality from someone, but we can give away our vitality by trying to get our way at the expense of the relationship. Do not blame the other person for the way you feel, changing their behavior will not solve your challenges with boundaries. If you have certain needs that are being fulfilled by a depleting relationship, identify them and determine if you can fulfill them in alternative ways. Consider receiving massage, painting, drawing or journaling. All of these activities can help you access your heart.

If your relationships are painful, recognize that pain is only a warning signal that something needs to change. If we don't heed the warning, then the pain will get more intense until we are forced to pay attention. Spend time in nature and set time aside daily to be in silence so that you can connect to your inner signals. While in connection with these signals you will naturally trust that your soul is guiding you to greater truth, wisdom, peace, and love.

I am aware of how I avoid pain, deny anger, and evading my fears. This depletes me so I choose to allow pain, acknowledge anger and accept my fears.

In every problem is its solution. Just like pain is a warning signal, the messages of comfort and discomfort in your relationships will guide you towards what you are not dealing with in your life. As our lives are primarily focused on increasing pleasure and avoiding pain, when we experience discomfort we often wall off our emotional pain. For example if you were teased as a kid you would learn not to show your pain because it would make you more vulnerable.

Anytime we constrict one emotion it hinders all our emotions and invisibly stops us from being vital. When an appropriate outlet for your emotions is unavailable, these destructive emotions are turned inward. For example in depression you feel hurt, but the expression of pain and anger are too great for you at the time so you turn these feelings against yourself. This arises when we don't know how to set an appropriate boundary. Fear can arise when you feel betrayed, but you are concerned that an appropriate boundary will lead to abandonment. Establishing clear boundaries with our loved ones is important otherwise we will hide our emotions so that we don't have to deal with them.

I embrace my uncomfortable and negative feelings, which enhances my capacity to experience the full depth and range of my vitalizing emotions.

Life is composed of opposites: hot and cold, wet and dry, mobile and stable. Without one we cannot have the other. This is true of our emotions as well. Without fear there cannot be love, without anger there cannot be joy. By embracing all of our emotions without judgment we open ourselves to wholehearted living. Our ecstasy is equal to our sorrow. The wound is the womb. When we acknowledge our multifaceted magnificence there is recognition that all of life is sacred. Even our selfish tendencies can lead to a fuller expression of generosity when embraced. When we experience our vulnerability and insecurity, we receive access to our courage and confidence. By opening ourselves to the full depth of our emotions we expand our capacity for vitality.

METABOLIZE YOUR FEELINGS

During the cleanse it is common for uncomfortable emotions to arise. When this occurs please follow the steps below to be able to work with these experiences in a productive way.

Describe what you are feeling while emotionally activated.

In describing your feelings as though you were a witness, you are able to determine whether you feel hurt, invalidated, unappreciated, angry, disappointed, invaded, neglected, taken advantage of, abandoned, or betrayed. In recognizing your response and becoming conscious of your emotional reactions, you will notice that you express a limited set of responses. By describing these, it will bring to light the limited range of responses regardless of the people who trigger you. Write them down so that you have a label to work within the following steps.

Identify where you feel the emotion in your body.

Once you have identified the feeling and described it attend to the experience in your body. Is there one area of your body that is generating the feelings? Is there more than one area? Once you have identified a primary area of the body that is involved, allow yourself to fully experience the sensations without attempting to resist or filter.

Express your emotional energy in beneficial ways.

Depending on where you experience the emotions, find a way to express it physically. Breathe, dance, sing, write, jump, laugh, roll around. Do whatever feels like it will release the stagnant energy. The key to making a beneficial change in your emotional patterns is your ability to witness the agitation, but not be overwhelmed by it. Physical expression allows the agitation to dissipate, accelerating the recovery of our emotional balance.

Explore why this incident triggered you.

Once you have physically expressed the emotional energy, begin to explore what it was about the situation that emotionally triggered you. Was it the words chosen, tone of voice, or body language? There are many subtle cues that are part of communication and they can transmit signals of appreciation or rejection, respect or threat. When we are emotionally triggered it is because of the inner tangle of memory and experience. Explore the situation by writing about the underlying cues that lead to your hurt feelings and be open to the hidden associations that arise.

Translate your emotional insights into love, safety, and intimacy.

By performing the activities above, you become more aware of your tendencies. As your internal dialogue determines your reality, understanding this dialogue can help you become responsible for your reality. With practice in metabolizing your feelings, you no longer waste energy by defending your territory. When you are less defensive, you learn to avoid your emotional landmines.

Yoga for Cleansing

The basic approach to yoga for cleansing is to do short sequences, about 20 minutes long, and to use the body movements as a platform for increased self-awareness. As you practice become aware of where you hold tension in the body. Is it the neck, the shoulders, the back? As you become more embodied and aware of what is taking place in your body then you can consciously allow the tension in your body to melt away. As this tension melts the universal intelligence that is communicating becomes more apparent. Although the type of postures and the sequencing of postures is important they can only take you so far. The real gift of yoga for cleansing is cultivating the awareness of changes in the body over time so that you can have an experientially based determination of whether or not the practices that you have initiated as a part of this program or in any area of your life are creating more relaxation in the body or more tension. Ultimately through cultivating this depth of awareness you will begin to see things more clearly and cultivate the perspective that will lead to increased levels of happiness.

Meditation for Cleansing

Any style of meditation or sitting will enhance the overall benefits of the Re-solution program. These days, there are many styles and strategies to choose from. If you have never meditated before, here are some brief instructions:

- Find a comfortable seated position. Comfort is key. You can sit cross-legged or in a chair. You can have your back supported or you can sit upright. The first principle of meditation is to start in a comfortable position.

- Once you have found that position then scan your body and become hyper-aware of the contact that your body makes against the surface beneath you.

- Once you really feel your seat and the way you are sitting and have made any adjustments then you can close your eyes. I like to set a timer for twenty minutes. There are many apps for this and I use one called Enso. Try and keep still, but if you need to fidget that is fine. If you are curious how much longer then softly open your eyes and see how many minutes remain.

- While you are sitting there pay close attention to the sensations in your body and the thoughts. The ultimate goal of meditation is to become profoundly aware of your attention. Where you put your attention is what you grow in your life. If you place your attention on your garden it grows. The essence of meditation is to become aware of where your attention is and then to course correct if your attention continuously goes back to things that you don't want to grow in your life. I have also included some meditation CD's in the resources section.

Pantry New Year Re-solution Shopping List

Many of the recipes in this manual require that you have some common pantry items. Although this list is not exclusive to this program it will give you a sense of some common supplies that you may need to have available. If you tend to shop on the perimeter of the supermarket it is likely you will already have many of these. This is your master list and may have some items that are also on the lists for each individual phase.

MASTER SHOPPING LIST

Grains

- ☐ Gluten free oatmeal or steel cut oats
- ☐ Quinoa or Cannehua
- ☐ Brown or White rice
- ☐ Wild rice

Beans

- ☐ Aduki beans
- ☐ Black beans
- ☐ French green lentils
- ☐ Split mung beans
- ☐ Pinto beans
- ☐ Red lentil

Nuts and Seeds

- ☐ Chia
- ☐ Flax
- ☐ Pumpkin
- ☐ Sesame
- ☐ Sunflower
- ☐ Hemp
- ☐ Hemp milk
- ☐ Shredded coconut
- ☐ Coconut milk

Oils

- ☐ Extra virgin sesame oil
- ☐ Extra virgin coconut oil
- ☐ Extra virgin olive oil
- ☐ Organic grass fed ghee

Condiments and Other

- ☐ Dijon Mustard
- ☐ Tamari (wheat free soy sauce)
- ☐ Baking soda

Herbs and Spices

- ☐ Ginger
- ☐ Garlic
- ☐ Cilantro
- ☐ Cumin
- ☐ Coriander
- ☐ Fennel
- ☐ Cinnamon
- ☐ Nutmeg
- ☐ Cardamom
- ☐ Turmeric
- ☐ Fenugreek
- ☐ Chili powder
- ☐ Curry powder
- ☐ Italian seasoning
- ☐ Basil
- ☐ Rosemary
- ☐ Tarragon
- ☐ Oregano
- ☐ Nutritional yeast

Sweeteners

- ☐ Stevia
- ☐ Honey

REMOVAL PHASE SHOPPING LIST
Vegetables

- ☐ 4–6 beets
- ☐ Spinach
- ☐ Zucchini
- ☐ Sweet potato
- ☐ Chard
- ☐ Fresh basil
- ☐ Onion
- ☐ Garlic
- ☐ Parsnips
- ☐ Turnips
- ☐ Celery
- ☐ Cabbage
- ☐ Cilantro
- ☐ Red pepper
- ☐ Parsley
- ☐ Green onion
- ☐ Avocado

Fruits

- ☐ 1 pint apple cider vinegar
- ☐ 4 lemons
- ☐ 1–2 pints of berries of your choice
- ☐ Raisins
- ☐ Lime
- ☐ Granny smith apples
- ☐ Grated coconut

Spices

- ☐ Powdered ginger
- ☐ Fresh ginger
- ☐ Cinnamon
- ☐ Cardamom
- ☐ Nutmeg
- ☐ Fennel powder
- ☐ Thyme
- ☐ Curry powder
- ☐ Chili powder
- ☐ Coriander powder
- ☐ Fenugreek powder
- ☐ Turmeric powder
- ☐ Cumin powder

Nuts and Seeds

- ☐ Flax seed
- ☐ Hemp or coconut milk
- ☐ Pumpkin seeds
- ☐ Hemp seeds

Oils

- ☐ Coconut oil
- ☐ Ghee
- ☐ Olive oil

Grains and Flours

- ☐ Coconut flour
- ☐ Wild rice

Beans

- ☐ Red lentils or split mung beans

Other

- ☐ Baking soda
- ☐ Psyllium husk powder
- ☐ Mustard
- ☐ Tamari
- ☐ Nutritional yeast
- ☐ Miso
- ☐ Dulse
- ☐ Honey

REPLACEMENT PHASE SHOPPING LIST

Tea

- ☐ Rooibos chai
- ☐ Kava Stress Relief
- ☐ Tension Tamer
- ☐ Vegetables
- ☐ Delicata squash
- ☐ Onion
- ☐ Garlic
- ☐ Shallot
- ☐ Kale
- ☐ Cauliflower
- ☐ Yam
- ☐ Fresh ginger
- ☐ Celery
- ☐ Carrot
- ☐ Potato
- ☐ Butternut squash
- ☐ Kale

Fruit

- ☐ Lemon
- ☐ Oranges

Spices

- ☐ Cardamom
- ☐ Cinnamon
- ☐ Ginger powder
- ☐ Oregano
- ☐ Nutmeg
- ☐ Turmeric
- ☐ Fresh rosemary
- ☐ Italian spice

Oil

- ☐ Ghee
- ☐ Coconut oil
- ☐ Olive oil

Nuts and Seeds

- ☐ Coconut milk
- ☐ Sunflower seed butter
- ☐ Sesame seeds

Other

- ☐ Vanilla crème liquid stevia
- ☐ Ashwagandha or Maca powder
- ☐ Dandy Blend coffee substitute
- ☐ Vanilla extract
- ☐ Rapunzel Vegetable bouillon
- ☐ Dijon mustard
- ☐ White wine vinegar
- ☐ Balsamic vinegar

LIQUID DIET DAY

Nuts and Seeds

- ☐ Hemp seeds
- ☐ Almonds

Vegetables

- ☐ Onion
- ☐ Fennel bulb
- ☐ Sweet potato
- ☐ Parsley
- ☐ Fresh ginger
- ☐ Cilantro
- ☐ Celery
- ☐ Zucchini
- ☐ Green leafy vegetables
- ☐ Parsley

Beans

- ☐ Chickpeas
- ☐ Split peas or whole mung beans

Oil

- ☐ Sesame oil

Fruits

- ☐ Dates

Grains and Flour

- ☐ Coconut flour

Spices

- ☐ Chili powder
- ☐ Curry powder
- ☐ Cinnamon
- ☐ Italian seasoning
- ☐ Coriander

Repair Phase Shopping List

Grains

- ☐ Basmati rice
- ☐ Quinoa

Beans

- ☐ Mung beans
- ☐ Split mung beans

Spices

- ☐ Curry powder
- ☐ Turmeric
- ☐ Black mustard seeds
- ☐ Cumin seeds
- ☐ Fennel seed
- ☐ Cardamom
- ☐ Clove
- ☐ Oregano
- ☐ Basil
- ☐ Bay leaves
- ☐ Black pepper
- ☐ Cayenne

Vegetables

- ☐ Cilantro
- ☐ Green leafy vegetables
- ☐ Fresh ginger
- ☐ Burdock root
- ☐ Parsnip root
- ☐ Broccoli raab
- ☐ Sweet potato
- ☐ Carrot
- ☐ Celery
- ☐ Red pepper
- ☐ Chard
- ☐ Tomato
- ☐ Fresh basil
- ☐ Shitake mushrooms
- ☐ Thai basil
- ☐ See Optional veggies
- ☐ Cabbage

Fruit

- ☐ Raisins
- ☐ Fresh berries
- ☐ Lime

Oils

- ☐ Ghee
- ☐ Coconut oil

Nuts and seeds

- ☐ Seed milk
- ☐ Coconut milk

Post Phase Shopping List

Dairy

- ☐ Nancy's Yogurt or Goat Yogurt
- ☐ Coconut milk

Spices

- ☐ Cinnamon powder
- ☐ Fennel powder
- ☐ Cardamom powder
- ☐ Cumin powder
- ☐ Coriander powder
- ☐ Cumin seed
- ☐ Coriander seed
- ☐ Fennel seed
- ☐ Licorice powder
- ☐ Vanilla extract
- ☐ Madras curry powder

Beans

- ☐ Red lentils

Seeds

- ☐ Chia seed
- ☐ Flax seed
- ☐ Sesame seed
- ☐ Sunflower seed

Vegetables

- ☐ Sweet potato
- ☐ Onion
- ☐ Garlic
- ☐ Tomato
- ☐ Shiitake mushroom
- ☐ Carrots
- ☐ Zucchini
- ☐ Bok choy
- ☐ Cilantro
- ☐ Shallot

Fruit

- ☐ Fuji apple
- ☐ Blueberries
- ☐ Strawberries
- ☐ Lemon
- ☐ Lime

Oil

- ☐ Coconut oil

Other

- ☐ Stevia
- ☐ Probiotic capsules
- ☐ Tamari

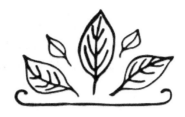

MORE RECIPES

General Recipe Suggestions for All Phases

Water Sauté: Instead of sautéing vegetables in oil, you can bring a small amount of water to a boil in a saucepan and add vegetables. You may have to add more water if the vegetables stick.

Pureed Vegetable Soups: For these soups, sauté onion, carrots and celery in water. Add a few seasonal vegetables, such as spinach, kale, chard, zucchini, parsnip, yams, broccoli, rutabaga, etc. You can also add seeds, such as sesame, pumpkin, sunflower, or hemp for protein. Fill the soup pot with enough water or vegetable stock to cover the veggies, put a lid on the pot, and bring to a boil. Reduce the heat and cook until the vegetables are tender. You can spice the soup with whatever spices you would like. Some suggestions are lemon, ginger, salt, coriander, and black pepper. Try broccoli soup, spinach soup, carrot ginger soup, and others.

Vegetable Bouillon: Place a cube of bouillon in rice, quinoa, amaranth, forbidden rice, wild rice, teff, or dahl for added flavor.

How to use Greens: Lightly steam or water sauté greens such as kale, chard, and spinach. Add lemon juice or soaked dried cranberries and raisins to sweeten them. Add sprouts or microgreens for an extra boost.

Mashes: Any root vegetables: parsnip, rutabaga, potato, daikon radish. Cut into cubes, boil until soft, and flavor with fresh rosemary.

Steamers: Steam broccoli, cauliflower, cabbage, carrots, bok choy, green beans, bell peppers, and asparagus; then season with lemon, salt, and coriander.

Salads: Salads may be made in a number of ways, including: mixed green salad; carrot salad; beet and apple salad; or cucumber salad with a dressing made of juice of one lemon, cilantro, avocado, salt, and fresh ginger.

Snacks: Sugar snap peas, rice cakes with apple butter, grapefruit, pears, carrot sticks with sunflower seed butter, celery sticks with pumpkin seed butter, rice cakes with yam butter, or rice cakes with bean pate.

TEA RECIPES

DIGESTIVE TEA

Ingredients:

- 1 teaspoon of fennel seed
- ½ teaspoon of coriander seed
- ¼ teaspoon of cumin seed
- 8 cups of water

Directions:

Boil for ten minutes strain and serve.

You can make a large pot and reheat it throughout the day.

Use more fennel and coriander seed if you like a slightly sweeter flavor.

You may also use any other kind of Detox tea that you like.

Checklist

	Phase	Remove			Replace				Repair				Post Phase			
	Day of the week	S	Sn	M	T	W	Th	F	S	Sn	M	T	W	Th	F	S
	Number	1	2	3	4	5	6	7	8	9	10	11	12	13	14	
Home Wellness guidelines																
	Three meals															
	Water intake in ounces															
	Self-massage															
	Steam or shower															
	Yoga															
	Breathwork															
	Meditation															
	Hydration therapy															
Daily Routines																
	Rising time															
	CCF tea															
	Lunch time															
	Bed time															
	Recapitulation															
Before every meal																
Sweet ease	Blood sugar															
Pitta digest	Digestion															
After every meal																
Kidney F.	Lymph/Adrenal															
Immune	Bile/Liver															
Turmeric	Colon															
Shilajit	Energy															
Other /Evening:																
Triphala	Bowel															
Other:																

Blank Menu Plan

	Removal phase			Replace Phase			
DAY	1	2	3	4	5	6	7
DATE							
	B:	B:	B:	B:	B:	B:	B:
	L:	L:	L:	L:	L:	L:	L:
	D:	D:	D:	D:	D:	D:	D:

	Liquid Diet	Repair Phase				Post Phase	
DAY	8	9	10	11	12	13	14
DATE							
	PURGE	B:	B:	B:	B:	B:	B:
	L:	L:	L:	L:	L:	L:	L:
	D:	D:	D:	D:	D:	D:	D:

Sample Daily Schedule

	REMOVAL PHASE			REPLACE PHASE			
DAY	1	2	3	4	5	6	7
DATE							
	Wellness Guidelines, Daily Guidelines, Lemon Water, ACV Elixir, Colorful food	Wellness Guidelines, Daily Guidelines, Lemon Water, ACV Elixir, Colorful food	Wellness Guidelines, Daily Guidelines, Lemon Water, ACV Elixir, Colorful food	Self-massage, Steam Therapy, Morning Elixir Wellness Guidelines, Daily Guidelines	Self-massage, Steam Therapy, Morning Elixir Wellness Guidelines, Daily Guidelines	Self-massage, Steam Therapy, Morning Elixir Wellness Guidelines, Daily Guidelines	Self Massage, Wellness Guidelines, Daily Guidelines, Self-massage, Steam Therapy, Morning Elixir

	REPAIR PHASE				POST PHASE		
DAY	8	9	10	11	12	13	14
DATE							
	Liquid Diet, Wellness Guidelines, Daily Guidelines,	Kitchari 3X's a day, Wellness Guidelines, Daily Guidelines	Kitchari 3X's a day, Wellness Guidelines, Daily Guidelines	Kitchari 3X's a day, Wellness Guidelines, Daily Guidelines,	Kitchari 3X's a day, Wellness Guidelines, Daily Guidelir es	Takra, Green leafy vegetables, gomasio seed powder, Wellness Guidelines, Daily Guideline Increase digestive herbs	Takra, Green leafy vegetables, gomasio seed powder, Wellness Guidelines, Daily Guidelines Increase digestive herbs

	Post Cleanse
DAY	14
DATE	
	Simple foods, Wellness Guidelines, Daily Guidelines

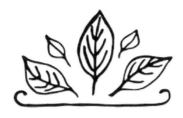

RESOURCES

THIS IS A SECTION DEVOTED TO FINDING THE SPECIFIC PRODUCTS THAT are recommended throughout the book and some guidelines on where to buy hard to find ingredients for some of the recipes.

Banyan Botanicals Ayurvedic Herbs

HERBAL TABLETS

Pitta Digest http://goo.gl/9vvRcR
Kapha Digest http://goo.gl/rg33Yv
Kidney Formula http://goo.gl/iN0Nca
Turmeric http://goo.gl/vXuxjj
Sweet Ease http://goo.gl/H968dr
Immune Support http://goo.gl/Z5COM2
Shilajit http://goo.gl/MEFoqN
Triphala http://goo.gl/e7JqRx

HERBAL OILS

4 oz Mahanarayan Oil http://goo.gl/TL2qQF

BULK HERBS AND SPICES

Ashwagandha http://goo.gl/dvT1xM
Shatavari http://goo.gl/mCbHWG
Amalaki http://goo.gl/NVQIvO

Tulsi http://goo.gl/UWTmvh
Guduchi http://goo.gl/yD7l1r
Licorice http://goo.gl/bNA5JG

Mountain Rose Herbs

BULK HERBS AND SPICES

Astragulus http://bit.ly/1L7n1eL
Schizandra http://bit.ly/1FvmKjn

Tools for Yoga

Yoga for Cleansing 3-DVD Set by Rhythm of Healing
http://bit.ly/1L7niON

Tools for Meditation

Best of Stress Management Kit by the Center for Mind-Body
Medicine www.cmbm.org
Meditation for Beginners by Jack Kornfield, includes a CD
Guided Mindfulness Mediation by Jon Kabat-Zin, Ph.D
Prana CD by Claudia Welch, DOM

Recommended Brands

Most of the recipes as part of this program require you to shop in the perimeter of the store. This means that most of what you will need can be found in the produce and bulk foods section of your favorite Natural Foods store. Some items however cannot be found in these areas and the below lists can be used as a guide of brands to consider purchasing.

Food Grade Oils

Big Tree Farms Barlean's Organic Oils Barleans.com
Costco's Kirkland Costco.com

McEvoy Ranch mcevoyranch.com

    Trader Joes' California Estate traderjoes.com

    Whole Food's 365 Everyday Value Unfiltered oils

        wholefoodsmarket.com

    Lucini Premium lucini.com

    Nutiva nutiva.com

    Living Harvest Livingharvest.com

    Spectrum Oil spectrum.com

Herbs and Spices

    Banyan Botanicals

    Mountain Rose Herbs

    Simply Organic

In the Kitchen

    Vitamix high speed blender Vitamix.com

    Xtrema Non toxic ceramic cookware Ceramcor.com

Teas

    Yogi Teas yogitea.com

    Organic India Tulsi Teas organicindiausa.com

    Dandy Blend Coffee Substitute

Get insider access to additional content and resources here: http://www.rhythmofhealing.com/newyearre-solution.html

Full Disclosure: *Many of the links above are affiliate links and I will receive a small commission, almost enough to buy a cup of tea when you purchase from these sites.*

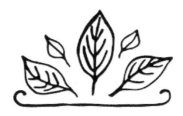

NOTES

Why Re-solution

1. Centers for Disease Control. Fourth National Report on Human Exposure to Environmental Chemicals. www.cdc.gov/exposurereport/pdf Fourth Report-Executive Summa pdf

2. United States Environmental Protection Agency, Toxics Release Inventory Program www.epa.gov/TRI

3. C. Pelletier P Imbeault, and A. Tremblay Energy Balance and Pollution by organochlorines and Polychlorinated Biphenyl obesity Reviews 4, no. 1 (2003) 17–24 A. Tremblay, C. Pelletier, E.

4. Environmental Working Group. Bisphenol A. www.ewg.org/chemind bisphenol A chemicals/

5. Environmental Gr Working Human Toxome Project, Mapping the Pollution in People. www. sites/humantoxome

6. Environmental Working Group. Pharmaceuticals pollute tapwater. ww node/ 6128

7. Gershon MD. 5-HT (Serotonin) physiology and related drugs. Curr Opin Gastroenterol 2000; 16: 113–20.Do 2. Herron, Fagan. Alternative Therapies in Health and Medicine, September/October 2002.

8. Sharma HM, Nidich S, Sands D, Smith DE. Improvement in cardiovascular risk factors through Panchakarma purification procedures. Journal of Research and Education in Indian Medicine, 1993, XI: 4, 2–13.

9. Nidich SI, Smith DE, Sands D, Sharma H. Nidich RJ, Barnes V, Jossang S. Effect of Maharishi Ayur-Ved karma purification program on speed of processing ability. Maharishi International University, Fairfield, Iowa, USA.

10. Panchakarma therapy greatly reduces the levels of 14 important 'lipophilic (i.e. fat-soluble) toxic and carcinogenic chemicals in the body.

11. Schneider RH Cavanaugh KL, Kasture HS, Rothenberg S, Averbach R, Robinson D, Wallace RK. Health promotion with a traditional system of natural health care: Maharishi Ayur-Veda. Journal of Social Behavior and Personality, 1990, 53): 1–2

Re-solution and Cleansing

12. Wilders-Truschnig, M., et al. 2007 IgE antibodies against food antigens are correlated with inflammation and intima media thickness in obese juveniles. Exp Clin Endocrinal Diabetes 116 (4):241–45

13. MacDonald, T>T., and G. Monteleone. 2005 Immunity, inflammation and allergy in the gut. Science 307:1920–1925

14. Atkinson, W., et al. 2007. Food elimination based on IgG antibodies in irritable bowel syndrome: A randomized controlled trial. Gut 53 (10):1459–1464

15. Susan J. Torres and Caryl A Nowson. Relationship between stress, eating behavior and obesity. Nutrition 2007:23:887–894

16. Linda Witek-Janusek et al. Psychological stress, reduced NK cell activity, and cytokine dysregulation in women experiencing diagnostic breast biopsy. Psychoneurondocrinology 2007;32:22–35

17. Mirjana Dimitrijevic et al. End-point effector stress mediators in neuroimmune interactions: their role in immune system homeostasis and autoimmune pathology Immunol Res, DOI 10.1007/s12026–012–8275–9

18. Y Tache and S. Brunnhuber. From Hans Selves discovery of bio-logical stress to the identification of corticotropin-releasing factor signaling pathways: implication in stress-related functional bowel diseases.

19. Sharma HM, Nidich S, Sands D, Smith DE. Improvement in cardio-vascular risk factors through Panchakarma purification proce-dures. Journal of Research and Education in Indian Medicine, 1993, XI: 4, 2–13.

20. Nidich SI, Smith DE, Sands D, Sharma H. Nidich RJ, Barnes V, Jos-sang S. Effect of Maharishi Ayur-Ved karma purification program on speed of processing ability. Maharishi International University, Fairfield, Iowa, USA.

21. Panchakarma therapy greatly reduces the levels of 14 important 'lipophilic (i.e. fat-soluble) toxic and carcinogenic chemicals in the body.

22. Schneider RH Cavanaugh KL, Kasture HS, Rothenberg S, Averbach R, Robinson D, Wallace RK. Health promotion with a traditional system of natural health care: Maharishi Ayur-Veda. Journal of Social Behavior and Personality, 1990, 53): 1–2

How to Prepare for a Successful Re-solution for Health

23. Leaching of aluminum from aluminum dishes and packages. Liukkonen-Lilja H, Piepponen S. Food Addit Contam. 1992 May-Jun;9(3):213–23. PMID: 1397396

24. Hesperidin and Silibinin Ameliorate **Aluminum**-Induced Neuro-toxicity: Modulation of Antioxidants and Inflammatory Cytokines Level in Mice Hippocampus. Jangra A, Kasbe P, Pandey SN, Dwivedi S, Gurjar SS, Kwatra M, Mishra M, Venu AK, Sulakhiya K, Gogoi R, Sarma N, Bezbaruah BK, Lahkar M. Biol Trace Elem Res. 2015 May 28. [Epub ahead of print]PMID: 26018497

25. Fourth National Report on Human Exposure to Environmental Chemicals. Center for Disease Control.

26. www.cdc.gov/exposurereport/pdf/FourthReport_ExecutiveSummary.pdf

Ahara: General Dietary Recommendations

27. T Colin Campbell and Thomas M. Campbell, The China Study (BenBella Books Dallas, 2006)

28. E. T Poehlman, P J. Arciero, C. L. Melby, and S. F. Badylak, "Resting Metabolic Rate and Postprandial Thermogenesis in Vegetarians and Nonvegetarians American Journal of Clinical Nutrition 48, no. 2 (1988): 209–13

29. S. E. McCann, J. L. Fredenheim, J. R. Marshall, and S. Graham, "Risk of Human ovarian Cancer Is Related to Dietary Intake of Selected Nutrients, Phytochemicals and Food Groups Journal of Nutrition 133, no. 6 (2003): 1937–42

30. K. A. Steinmetz and J. D. Potter "Vegetables, Fruit and Cancer Prevention: A Review 1996 Journal of the American Dietetic Association 96, no. 10 1027–39

31. Y Papikolaou and V. L. Fulgoni, "Bean Consumption Is Associated with Greater Nutrient intake, Reduced Systolic Blood Pressure, Lower Body Weight, and a smaller waist Circumference in Adults": Results from the National Health and Nutrition Examination Survey 999–2002, Journal of the American College of Nutrition 27, no. 5 (2008): 569–76

32. F.B. Hu, J E. Manson, and W.C. Willett, "Types of Dietary Fat and Risk of Coronary Disease: A Critical Review," Journal of the American College of Nutrition 20, no (2001): 5–19

33. Leray C. 2010. Cyberlipid Center.: Resource site for lipid studies. Available from: http://www.cyberlipid.org/cyberlip/home0001.htm

34. Femke Lutgendorff Louis M. A. Akkermans, and Johan D. Soder-holm The role of microbiota and probiotics in stress-induced gastro-intestinal damage. Curr Mol Med 2008;8:282–298

35. Tapsell LC, Hemphill I, Cobiac L, Patch CS, Sullivan DR, Fenech M, Roodenrys S, Keogh JB, Clifton PM, Williams PG, Fazio VA, Inge KE. 2006. Health benefits of herbs and spices: the past, the present, the future. Med J Aust. 185(4 Suppl):S4–24

36. Yolanda Gonzalez et al. High glucose concentrations induce TNF-alpha production through the down-regulation of CD33 in primary human monocytes. BMC Immunology 2012; 13:19, DOI: 10.1186/1471 –2172–13–19 6.

37. Angel Gil-Izquierdo, Maria I. Gil, and Federico Ferreres, "Effect of Processing Techniques at Industrial Scale on Orange Juice Antiox-idant and Beneficial Health Compounds," Journal of Agricultural and Food Chemistry 50, no. 18 (2002): 5107–14

38. Deborah Rothman, Pamela DeLuca, and Robert B. Zurier. Botan-ical lipids: effects on inflammation, immune responses and rheu-matoid arthritis. Semi Arthritis Rheu 1995 Oct 25(2):87–96

39. Anna Sapone et al. Spectrum of gluten-related disorders: consen-sus on new nomclature and classification. BMC Medicine 2012; 10:13 2.

40. Paimela al. Gliadin immune reactivity in patient with rheumatoid arthritis. Clin et Exp Rheumatol 1995 Sep-Oct; 13(5):603–607 4.

41. Amy C. Brown. Gluten sensitivity: problems of an emerging condi-tion separate f celiac disease. Expert Rev Gastroenterol Hepatol 2012;6(1):43–55 5.

42. ParkerG, Crawford J. 2007. Chocolate craving when depressed: a personality marker. Br J Psychiatry. 191:351–2

General Home Wellness Guidelines

43. S.H. Holt, J. Miller, P. Petocz and Farmakalidis, A Satiety Index of Common Foods European Journal of Clinical Nutrition 49, no. 9 (1995): 675–90

44. R. J. Barnard, E. J. Ugianskis, D. A. Martin, and S. B. Ink, "Role of Diet and Exercise in the Management of Hyperinsulinemia Athero-sclerotic and Associate Risk Factors" American Journal of Cardiol-ogy 69, no. 5 (1992): 440–444

Using Herbs to Maximize your Benefits

45. Rasyid A Lelo A. The effect of curcumin and placebo on human gene function: an ultrasound study. Aliment Pharmacol Ther. 1999;13:245–249

46. Baskaran K et al. Antidiabetic effect of leaf extract from Gymnema sylvestre a in noninsulin-dependent diabetes mellitus patients. J Ethnopharmacoll990, 30:295

47. Shanmugasundaram ER. et al. Use of Gynmema sylvestre leaf extract in the control of blood glucose in insulin-dependent dia-betes mellitus. J Ethnopharmacoll990, 30:281

48. Visser SA. Effect of humic substances on mitochondrial respi-ration and oxidative phosphorylation. Sci Total Environ. 1987 Apr62:347–54.

49. Peat Ghosal UK: Narosa Publishing House 2006 s. Shilajit in Per-spective. Oxford, 7,8,9,10,11 12 clinical study for antioxidant capac-ity and safe use of purified and evaluation of plasma standard-ized Shilajit (RevitalET) in normal volunteers.

50. J. B. Roy State Ayurvedic Medical College and Hospital, Kolkata. 2007. Data on file. Natreon, Inc. 13. Paraquat Fischer, A.M, Win-terie, J.S., Mill, T. (1967). Primary photochemical processes in pho-tolysis medicated by humic substances. In R.G. zika, w J. Cooper (Eds).

ABOUT THE AUTHOR

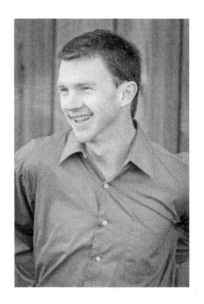

NOAH VOLZ IS THE OWNER OF RHYTHM of Healing an Ayurvedic clinic which emphasizes a personalized, mind-body approach to health. He is also the creator of the Yoga for Cleansing DVD. His mission is to protect ancient Ayurvedic wisdom and to support grassroots sustainable healthcare efforts across the world.

56610564R00114

Made in the USA
Columbia, SC
28 April 2019